Drugs and the Liver

Drugs and the Liver

A guide to drug handling
in liver dysfunction

Edited by
Penny North-Lewis

BPharm, MRPharmS, ClinDipPharm, MSc

Lead Paediatric Liver Pharmacist, Leeds Teaching Hospitals NHS Trust,
Leeds, UK

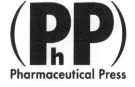
Pharmaceutical Press

Published by Pharmaceutical Press

1 Lambeth High Street, London SE1 7JN, UK

© Royal Pharmaceutical Society of Great Britian 2008

(**PP**) is a trade mark of Pharmaceutical Press
Pharmaceutical Press is the publishing division of the Royal Pharmaceutical Society

First edition published 2008
Reprinted 2011

Typeset by Photoprint, Torquay, Devon
Printed and bound by CPI Group (UK) Ltd, Croydon, CR0 4YY

ISBN 978 0 85369 710 7

A catalogue record for this book is available from the British Library.

Contents

Preface

It is well recognised that the majority of medicines pass through the liver on their journey around the body, but little is published on how different types and degrees of liver dysfunction affect the body's ability to handle those medicines. This is because clinical studies are typically conducted in small numbers of patients with a specific liver disease, usually classified generically as 'mild to moderate'. The results of these studies are often misguidedly extrapolated to all types of liver dysfunction. To exacerbate the problem, because of the scarcity of data, pharmaceutical companies frequently suggest dose reductions or the avoidance of a particular medicine in liver dysfunction. These effects combine to leave patients with liver disease disenfranchised from medicine use by the lack of information available to assist prescribers.

To make a judgement on medicine and choice of dose in an individual patient with a certain type of liver dysfunction, one must often return to first principles to make an educated guess. The aim of this book is therefore:

- To enable the practitioner to assess liver function using biochemical markers (e.g. liver function tests), other tests, signs, symptoms and disease knowledge
- To identify which pharmacokinetic and pharmacodynamic parameters of a drug are likely to be affected by different types of liver disease
- To consider the impact of a drug's side effects on a patient with liver disease.

This book is written by pharmacists and clinicians in the field of hepatology and is designed to assist practitioners to make these decisions. It is aimed primarily at clinical pharmacists, but may be of value to anyone making medicine choices in patients with liver impairment, as well as to students of pharmacokinetics. It is not aimed at academics and does not negate the need for further investigation, but it will enable practitioners to make pragmatic choices for their patients.

Penny North-Lewis
June 2007

About the editor

Penny North-Lewis graduated from Nottingham University in 1989 with a BPharm(Hons). She went on to complete the London School of Pharmacy Clinical Diploma in 1992, and a Master of Science in Clinical Pharmacy at Brighton University in 1998.

Penny has been working in the field of hepatology since 1993, when she became the first clinical pharmacist to work with the paediatric liver unit at King's College Hospital, London. She remained there until 1998, and, after a short period working in adult medicine, moved to Leeds in 2000 to establish the clinical pharmacy service for the new Paediatric Liver and GI Unit at St James's University Hospital, where she has remained ever since. Her role entails close liaison with the consultants, including participation in their daily ward rounds and attendance at out-patient clinics. She has also been closely involved with the development of guidelines for managing patients with liver disease.

Penny has been involved with a wide range of clinical studies in children with liver disease. These include several that relate to pharmacokinetics, in both liver disease and after liver transplantation. She has presented her research work and given lectures and workshops at national and international congresses, including the International Pediatric Transplant Association, the European Society of Clinical Pharmacy and the Neonatal and Paediatric Pharmacists Group (NPPG) conferences.

She is a founder member of the UK and Eire Liver Transplant Pharmacists Group, which was set up in 1994 to provide pharmacists in this field with the opportunity to learn, share ideas and help solve problems. She is also on the committee of the NPPG.

Contributors

Michael Bowe, BPharm, MRPharmS, ClinDipPharm
Lead GI and Liver Pharmacist (at the time of writing)
Pharmacy Department, Freeman Hospital
Newcastle-upon-Tyne, UK

Faye Croxen, BPharm, MRPharmS, ClinDipPharm
Lead Adult Liver Pharmacist
Pharmacy Department, Leeds Teaching Hospitals NHS Trust
Leeds, UK

Bridget Featherstone, BSc(Hons), MRPharmS, DipClinPharm, SP
Lead Pharmacist Transplantation and Surgery
Pharmacy Department, Cambridge University Teaching Hospitals
NHS Trust, Cambridge, UK

Kylies Foot, BPharm(Hons) (University of South Australia), MRPharmS
Liver Specialist Medicines Information Pharmacist (at the time of writing)
Medicines Information Centre, Pharmacy Department
Leeds Teaching Hospitals NHS Trust
Leeds, UK

Andrew Holt, MBChB(Hons), MRCP
Honorary Clinical Fellow in Hepatology
Liver Research Laboratory, MRC Centre for Immune Regulation
University of Birmingham, UK

Catherine Hughes, BPharm(Hons), MRPharmS, DipClinPharm
Lead Adult Liver Pharmacist (at the time of writing)
Pharmacy Department, Leeds Teaching Hospitals NHS Trust
Leeds, UK

Trevor N Johnson, BPharm, MSc, PhD, MRPharmS, MCPP
Senior Pharmacist, Pharmacy Department, Sheffield Children's
Hospital and Senior Scientist, Simcyp Limited
Sheffield, UK

Fionnuala Kennedy, BSc(Pharm), BA(Econ), MA(Healthcare Manag), MPSI
Clinical Pharmacy Manager/Lead Liver Pharmacist
Pharmacy Department, St Vincent's University Hospital
Dublin, Ireland

Sarah Knighton, MPharm, MRPharmS, DipClinPharm
Liver Pharmacy Team Leader
Pharmacy Department, King's College Hospital
London, UK

Saw Keng Lee, MPharm, MRPharmS, DipPharmPrac
Senior Liver Pharmacist (at the time of writing)
Pharmacy Department, King's College Hospital
London, UK

Penny North-Lewis, BPharm, MRPharmS, DipClinPharm, MSc
Lead Paediatric Liver Pharmacist
Pharmacy Department, Leeds Teaching Hospitals NHS Trust
Leeds, UK

Aileen Parke, MRPharmS, SP, MSc
Women and Children's Pharmacy Team Leader
Pharmacy Department
King's College Hospital
London, UK

Amanda Smith, BPharm, MRPharmS, DipClinPharm
Lead Pharmacist, Liver and Solid Organ Transplantation
Pharmacy Department, University Hospital Birmingham NHS
Foundation Trust
Birmingham, UK

Alison H Thomson, MSc, PhD, MRPharmS, MCPP
Area Pharmacy Specialist, Western Infirmary and Senior Lecturer
Strathclyde Institute of Pharmacy and Biomedical Sciences, University
of Strathclyde
Glasgow, UK

**Janet Tweed, BPharm, MRPharmS, DipClinPharm, Certificate in
Pharmaceutical Information Management**
Medicines Information Service Development Manager
Medicines Information Centre, Pharmacy Department
Leeds Teaching Hospitals NHS Trust
Leeds, UK

**Sheetal (Tina) Vaghjiani, BSc(Hons)Pharm, MRPharmS,
DipClinPharm**
Senior Pharmacist – Hepatology, Gastroenterology and Nutrition
Pharmacy Department, Royal Free Hampstead NHS Trust
London, UK

Acknowledgements

This book could not have been written without the enormous commitment of my fellow collaborators in the UK and Eire Liver Transplant Pharmacists Group. My thanks go to every member for their role in ensuring this goal has been realised. I would especially like to extend my thanks to Katherine Davidson for reviewing chapters with a fresh eye, to Helen Whiteside for helping at the planning stage, to Janet Tweed (nee Darlington) for being unstintingly conscientious despite staffing shortages and getting married, to Catherine Hughes for being endlessly supportive, and to Richard Coverdale for project managing me. I am also indebted to Professor Liz Kay for allowing me and others at Leeds Teaching Hospitals the time and resources to complete this project, to all the medical colleagues involved for their interest, support and assistance in reviewing each chapter in the book, and the staff at Pharmaceutical Press for their patience and support.

Introduction

How to use the book

In order to understand the extent of a patient's liver dysfunction you need to understand how the liver works and what it does. If you are unfamiliar with hepatology you should read Chapters 1 and 2, which provide an outline of normal anatomy, physiology and functions of the liver. They enable you to visualise how blood moves around the liver and so understand the implications of a portal vein thrombosis; to understand hepatocyte function, which helps explain why your patient has coagulopathy; to imagine how bile flows and the pathophysiology of gallstones. You may not need to refer to it again, but it is a useful resource if you are confronted with something you have not come across before.

Once you have grasped the basics of hepatology, Chapter 3 gives examples of some of the more common liver diseases seen in adults and children, and highlights what changes they make to the liver's metabolic/eliminative function. There are hundreds of liver diseases, but we have only mentioned the most common: the Further Reading section gives recommendations for where to find more information about specific diseases not discussed here.

Chapter 4 guides you in understanding how a patient's signs and symptoms of liver disease, coupled with liver function and other laboratory or diagnostic tests, give an indication of the severity of the liver dysfunction.

Having assessed liver function, you need to go back to basic principles of pharmacokinetics: what does the liver normally do and what types of dysfunction may affect drug handling? In Chapter 5 we have incorporated the theory with practical advice that you can apply to a patient. Chapter 6 considers the impact of a drug's side-effect profile on a patient with liver dysfunction.

This is a practical guide rather than a scientific tome, finishing in Part 3 with worked examples of commonly asked questions: which analgesic should you recommend for a patient with acute liver failure? What is the best lipid-lowering agent for someone with chronic liver disease? The idea of this section is also to guide you through the questions you need to ask to be able to answer the more unusual queries for yourself – going back to first principles of assessing liver function and drug pharmacokinetics. It is not possible to give an answer to the question of whether or not a particular drug can be used in a patient with liver disease because everything depends on the patient in front of you, and there are too many possible permutations. The *aide mémoire* is a tool to help you remember which aspects of the patient and the drug you need to be especially aware of.

This is our first attempt at providing a practical method to help pharmacists answer questions about drug use in this group of patients. It illustrates the way in which experienced liver pharmacists deal with these problems and distils our experience into a user-friendly form. I welcome any feedback on the approach taken in this book.

Part One

Understanding liver function

1

An introduction to the anatomy of the liver

Andrew Holt and Amanda Smith

Objectives

This chapter will help you understand:

- The basic anatomy and function of the liver.
- Hepatocyte function and the role of other cells in the human liver.
- The functional anatomy of the biliary tree.

Introduction

The liver is the largest solid organ in the human body, weighing approximately 1.6 kg in men and 1.4 kg in women, and comprises 2% of adult body weight. Anatomically it is located under the diaphragm in the right upper quadrant of the abdomen, protected anteriorly and posteriorly by the rib cage. It has two lobes, the right lobe being six times larger than the left.

The liver is a highly vascular structure which receives approximately 1.3 L of blood each minute. The blood supply originates from two sources: 75% is provided by the portal vein, which drains the gut, and the remainder is provided by the hepatic artery, which originates at the coeliac plexus of the aorta. These two blood supplies combine to provide the nutrient- and oxygen-rich blood necessary for the metabolic processes that occur in liver tissue. As a consequence the liver is perfectly placed within the circulation to gather and process metabolites and to eliminate toxins.

Liver tissue is composed predominantly of cells called hepatocytes, which occupy 80–88% of the total liver volume in humans. Hepatocytes and other liver cells perform vital functions, such as

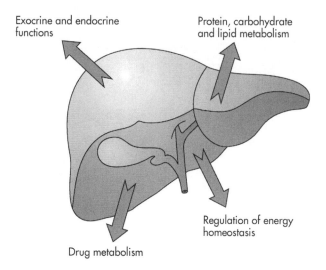

Exocrine and endocrine functions

Protein, carbohydrate and lipid metabolism

Regulation of energy homeostasis

Drug metabolism

Figure 1.1 Functions of the liver.

protein synthesis and regulation of energy homoeostasis, which maintain the health of an individual and support the function of many other organ systems. In addition, the liver supervises the metabolism and excretion of many drugs and toxins while providing an immune barrier to pathogens and antigens transported via the portal vein. Because of its importance in these metabolic processes, decisions to prescribe in patients with hepatic dysfunction must take into account the capacity of the liver to metabolise drugs successfully (Figure 1.1).

Embryology

The liver appears in the third week of gestation as an outgrowth of pluripotent cells in the region that will become the duodenum. These cells differentiate into tissues that will ultimately become the liver, biliary tree and gallbladder. By the fourth week the liver has already developed a system of tiny blood vessels or sinusoids arranged around the hepatocytes, reflecting the vascular structure of the adult liver. Simultaneously the biliary tree develops, and can be identified by the sixth week of gestation as a series of tiny biliary canaliculi and a primitive extrahepatic biliary tree; the flow of bile begins by the third month.

The liver grows quickly, accounting for 10% of foetal mass by the 10th week. This is largely due to the number of newly formed sinusoids, but another important factor is the haematopoietic function of the embryonic liver, which is responsible for foetal blood production from the end of the first month of gestation. This haematopoietic activity subsides during the last 8 weeks of intrauterine life as the bone marrow assumes this role [1]. At term, the liver constitutes about 5% of total body weight.

Despite its complexity, the liver is not a site associated with a significant number of congenital defects, although there are a considerable number of lobular, vascular and biliary anatomical variants described. For example, only 50% of the population have 'normal' biliary anatomy; the remainder possess subtle variations which are important to recognise when planning surgery [2]. The comparative rarity of serious congenital defects may reflect their lethal nature, resulting in spontaneous abortion at a very early stage of embryogenesis. Some babies are born with biliary defects or present with jaundice in the postnatal period. Biliary atresia, a condition where the extrahepatic biliary tree fails to develop, causes neonatal conjugated hyperbilirubinaemia, and may be associated with other anatomical defects. Early surgical intervention in the form of the Kasai procedure or liver transplantation has radically improved the prognosis of this once fatal disease [3].

Anatomy

Gross anatomy of the liver

The liver is found underneath the ribs in the right upper quadrant of the abdomen, close to other organs such as the lungs and pleura, which are separated from the liver by the diaphragm. The right kidney and hepatic flexure of the transverse colon lie slightly behind the right lobe of the liver, with the stomach overlying the left lobe. During inspiration the liver moves in sympathy with the diaphragm, allowing it to be palpated through the anterior abdominal wall. The tip of the gallbladder sometimes protrudes below the liver and may also be felt if it becomes grossly enlarged. A thorough knowledge of the relationships of the liver to surrounding structures is very important when performing procedures such as liver biopsy or paracentesis, to prevent injury to neighbouring tissues (Figure 1.2).

In health the liver is a large smooth organ covered in a protective cellophane-like membrane known as Glisson's capsule. This thin layer of connective tissue becomes thicker around the hilum, where the portal vein and hepatic artery enter the liver and where the right and left hepatic ducts and lymphatics exit. The surface of the liver is broadly

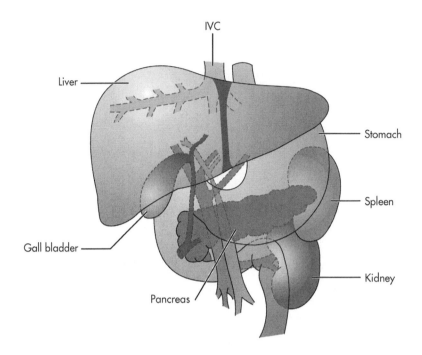

IVC

Liver

Stomach

Spleen

Gall bladder

Kidney

Pancreas

Figure 1.2 Anatomical position of the liver.

divided into two lobes by the falciform ligament. Although this appears to divide the liver into two, in fact it has no functional significance other than to attach the liver to the diaphragm and anterior abdominal wall. The physiological division of the liver into right and left lobes follows the partition of the portal vein into its main right and left branches. This can be visualised on the surface of the liver by drawing an imaginary line from the tip of the gallbladder to the groove of the inferior vena cava (IVC).

Blood supply of the liver

Seventy-five percent of the blood received by the liver is venous and is supplied by the portal vein, which drains the capillary beds of the digestive tract, spleen, pancreas and gallbladder. Arterial blood is provided by the hepatic artery, which originates from the aorta and enters the liver alongside the portal vein. Once the portal vein enters the liver it divides into the right and left main branches and then subdivides to supply the various regions of the liver. The separation of the portal vein to supply the different liver sections provides a convenient means of

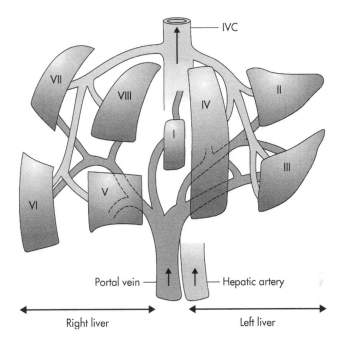

Figure 1.3 Segments of the liver.

subdividing the liver into eight smaller segments, as described by Couinaud [4], each being supplied by its own branch of the portal vein (Figure 1.3).

The left branch of the portal vein supplies segments 2, 3 and 4, and the right branch supplies segments 5, 6, 7 and 8. Segment 1 (or the caudate lobe) has its own blood supply from the portal vein and drains directly into the IVC. These segments do not have surface landmarks and are not physically separate within the liver, but identifying their boundaries enables surgeons to safely resect diseased liver tissue and allows donor livers to be split for transplantation where necessary. The hepatic artery is subdivided inside the liver into smaller branches which complement the divisions of the portal vein. Each segment of the liver drains blood back into the circulation through a series of veins that join to form three large hepatic veins; these ultimately drain into the IVC, which returns blood to the heart.

Large volumes of blood flow through the normal liver without interruption, but in many liver diseases vascular resistance is increased and the velocity of blood flow through the liver is slowed. In cirrhosis the small vessels and sinusoids become scarred, leading to an increase in resistance to blood flow and causing the pressure in the portal vein to rise (portal hypertension). The increased portal pressure promotes the formation of varices and ascites and may ultimately give rise to hepatorenal syndrome. Slowing of the portal venous blood flow also increases the risk of thromboses within the portal vein, which may exacerbate any deterioration in liver function.

Rarely blood flow may be interrupted at the level of the hepatic sinusoids in sinusoidal obstruction syndrome (veno-occlusive disease), leading to an acute deterioration in liver function. This unusual syndrome has many causes, including drugs, e.g. azathioprine, or chemotherapeutic conditioning regimens such as busulphan with cyclophosphamide. Obstruction of blood flow out of the liver (e.g. in Budd–Chiari syndrome) may also cause significant liver injury, and in cases where all three of the hepatic veins suddenly become blocked fulminant hepatic failure can occur, necessitating urgent liver transplantation or radiological stenting.

The liver lobule

There are several different ways to describe the cellular anatomy of the liver, the simplest of which is the view seen when the liver is examined under a light microscope (Figure 1.4).

High-power magnification reveals the hepatocytes arranged in rows of cells radiating out from a central vein like spokes in a wheel, forming polygonal regions called lobules. In other mammals, e.g. the pig, the lobules are separated by a layer of connective tissue, but in humans they are not segregated in this way, making it difficult to differentiate between adjacent lobules. At the corner of each lobule a collection of blood vessels (a branch of both the hepatic artery and portal vein) and a bile duct emerge from a sheath of connective tissue; this region is referred to as the portal tract (Figure 1.5).

The rows of hepatocytes are separated by blood-filled channels which anastomose freely to form a labyrinth of specialised capillaries, termed liver sinusoids. The liver sinusoids are highly adapted, designed to facilitate easy transfer of molecules from the lumen of the sinusoid to the hepatocytes, and vice versa. The endothelial cells that line the sinusoid are highly permeable as they lack a basement membrane and contain small holes (or fenestrations) within the cell, which perforate the cytoplasm and cluster together to form 'sieve plates'. Proteins and other molecules passing across the sinusoid percolate through the sieve plate and gaps between the cells into a space separating the endothelium

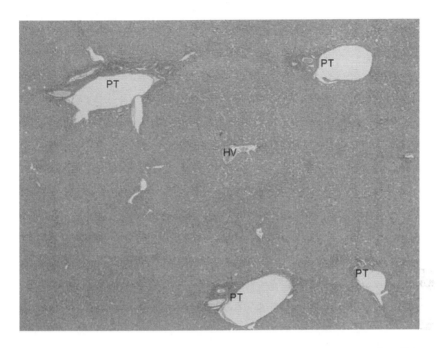

Figure 1.4 The classic liver lobule (Dr Desley Neil, Department of Cellular Pathology, University Hospital Birmingham NHS Foundation Trust).

and hepatocytes called the space of Disse. This gap between cells allows hepatocytes to be continuously bathed in plasma, facilitating rapid and efficient exchange of substrates and metabolites from the circulation to the hepatocyte, and vice versa.

The liver acinus

Although the classic lobular model describes the microscopic appearance of the liver well, a better way to understand how the liver functions is to subdivide it into regions of hepatocytes irrigated by a single portal tract – an area referred to as the hepatic acinus.

Blood emerging from the portal tract filters through the network of sinusoidal channels that separate rows of hepatocytes on its way towards the central vein. The hepatocytes within the acinus can be subdivided into three zones according to their distance from the portal venule. Cells in close proximity to the portal triad are the first to receive the nutrient- and oxygen-rich blood, and are consequently most

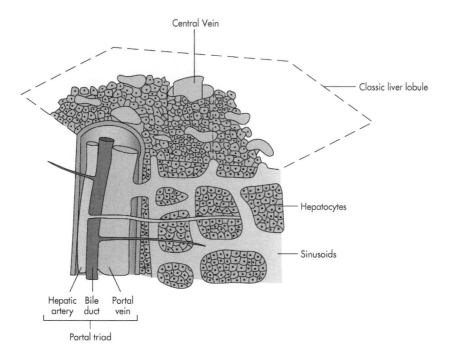

Central Vein

Classic liver lobule

Hepatocytes

Sinusoids

Hepatic Bile Portal
artery duct vein

Portal triad

Figure 1.5   Cross-section of a liver lobule.

resistant to ischaemic injury; this region is denoted zone 1. Hepatocytes further from the portal tract will receive blood with a lower concentration of nutrients; the most peripheral cells, in zone 3, are adjacent to the central vein and at greatest risk of hypoxic injury owing to the low oxygen tension of perivenular sinusoidal blood. This region corresponds to the central lobular zone of the classic liver lobule (Figure 1.6).

The distribution of metabolic functions within acinar zones is determined principally by the microenvironment of the hepatocytes. Cells in zone 1 are the first to respond to changes in the portal blood, such as glucose and insulin levels, and therefore play important roles in glycolysis and gluconeogenesis. Protein synthesis, β-oxidation of fatty acids, cholesterol synthesis and bile acid secretion also predominate in zone 1. Ordinarily zone 3 hepatocytes are the principal site of cytochrome P450 oxidation/reduction activity as well as NADPH and NADH reductase metabolism, making this region more susceptible

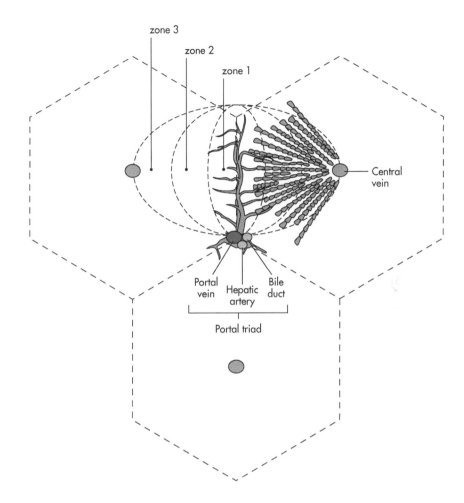

Figure 1.6 Liver acinus.

to drug-induced liver injury. Interestingly, reversing acinar blood flow in animal models and directing oxygen- and nutrient-rich blood to zone 3 hepatocytes stimulates 'zone 1' protein synthesis and glycolysis in these cells [5]. However, reversing acinar blood flow does not alter mixed function oxidation or glutamine synthase activity, suggesting that some metabolic functions operate under different control mechanisms, which may be genetically determined. This model is unable to explain all of the physiological complexity of the acinus, but does explain some of the different patterns of hepatocyte injury in various disease conditions, or as a consequence of different toxic agents.

Cellular biology of the liver

The hepatocyte

Liver cells are possibly the most versatile somatic cells in the entire body. Hepatocytes are the chief functional cells, possessing exocrine and endocrine properties in addition to performing a wide range of tasks such as protein synthesis, carbohydrate and lipid metabolism, and detoxification of drugs. They store energy in the form of sugar (glycogen) and fats (triglyceride), regulating and releasing energy from these stores between meals and during sleep. During fasting or in sickness the liver can convert amino acids and lipids into glucose by means of a complex catabolic enzymatic process termed gluconeogenesis. The liver also functions as the main site of amino acid deamination, via the urea cycle, resulting in urea which is eventually excreted from the kidney.

Hepatocytes constitute approximately 80% of the human liver, and lie arranged in plates around the sinusoids. These large polyhedral cells measure about 20–30 μm in diameter, have up to six surfaces, and are arranged in rows one or two hepatocytes thick along the sinusoids. A single hepatocyte can be in contact with several sinusoids as well as neighbouring hepatocytes. About 70% of the hepatocyte surface is in contact with sinusoids, separated from the endothelial cell by the space of Disse. This surface is covered by short microvilli, which increase the available surface area for transfer of various substances between the sinusoidal lumen and the cell. The remaining surfaces abut neighbouring hepatocytes, providing firm cellular attachment via tight junctions, and permitting cell-to-cell signalling across communicating junctions. Some of the surfaces between adjacent hepatocytes contain tiny channels about 0.5–2.5 μm in diameter called canaliculi. These are lined by irregular microvilli which facilitate the secretion of biliary constituents from the hepatocyte into the biliary tree. The cell membrane around the canaliculus is rich in alkaline phosphatase and ATP.

The functional diversity of the hepatocyte necessitates a large number of cytoplasmic organelles. Under electron microscopy hepatocytes possess many features that are characteristic of cells involved in a wide variety of metabolic functions, including numerous mitochondria, lysosomes, peroxisomes (or microbodies), rough and smooth endoplasmic reticulum, and glycogen stored within the cytoplasm (Figure 1.7).

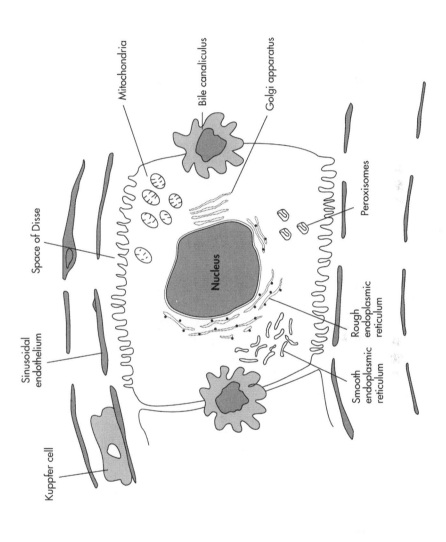

Figure 1.7 The hepatocyte.

Hepatocyte nucleus

Hepatocytes contain large nuclei which can occupy up to 10% of the cell volume. About 25% of hepatocytes are binucleate, and this proportion increases with age or following a stimulus to liver regeneration.

Mitochondria

Hepatocytes contain large numbers of mitochondria, which account for about 20% of cytoplasmic volume in the adult liver. These are required to meet the high energy demands of liver tissue, which they fulfil by producing ATP from pyruvate via the Krebs cycle. In addition to ATP synthesis, mitochondria are involved in a variety of other metabolic pathways, including fatty acid oxidation, steroid metabolism, nucleic acid synthesis, regulation of intracellular calcium levels and haem biosynthesis. Proteins associated with the mitochondrial membrane play a central role in the regulation and execution of programmed cell death, or apoptosis. As the liver ages the volume and shape of the mitochondria remain constant but their numbers appear to decrease.

Endoplasmic reticulum and the Golgi apparatus

The endoplasmic reticulum (ER) and Golgi apparatus are involved in the processing of proteins. These proteins are synthesised in the ER, transported to the Golgi apparatus and prepared for export or utilisation within the cell. Human hepatocytes possess an abundance of endoplasmic reticulum, both smooth and rough. The proportion of the two types varies among animal species, although in humans approximately three-quarters is of the smooth type. Rough ER is predominantly localised along the sinusoidal border of the hepatocyte, concentrated around the nucleus and mitochondria of the cell, and is the major site of protein synthesis. Proteins are transcribed from messenger RNA within saccular extrusions called ribosomes in readiness for export from the cell. Although some of the proteins secreted from the liver are derived from macrophages, over 90% of the protein produced by the liver is synthesised by hepatocytes, which export them from the cell into the bloodstream. All hepatocytes synthesise a wide variety of proteins, such as albumin, binding proteins for hormones and growth factors, and coagulation factors (fibrinogen, prothrombin).

In contrast to rough ER, smooth ER is dispersed throughout the hepatocytes and exists as collections of vesicles closely associated with aggregates of glycogen granules. Smooth ER is highly developed in hepatocytes and functions predominantly to synthesise lipid, accumulate and sequester glycogen, and metabolise drugs and steroids. To carry out these functions, the membrane of the smooth ER contains many important enzymes, such as NADPH-cytochrome-C reductase and cytochrome P450, which determine the biotransformation of drugs and endogenous steroids via the microsomal mono-oxygenase system. Induction of P450 by drugs is associated with an increase in the amount of smooth ER within the cell [6–8]. In addition, smooth ER contains enzymes involved in the synthesis of cholesterol, the formation of bile salts and the removal of iodine from thyroid hormones, and performs several important processes such as conjugation, where substances (e.g. bilirubin) are conjugated to sulphate or glucuronide moieties during inactivation or in preparation for excretion from the body. A specialised form of ER known as the Golgi apparatus is found in the vicinity of bile canaliculi. These structures are concerned with the assembly and packaging of lipoproteins (very low-density lipoprotein, VLDL), glycoproteins (e.g. transferrin) and plasma proteins (e.g. albumin) in readiness for export or incorporation into intracellular components.

Lysosomes and peroxisomes

Lysosomes are in effect a cellular waste-bin, and play an important role in the turnover and degradation of cytoplasmic organelles and phagocytosed particles. They facilitate receptor-mediated endocytosis of many macromolecules from the cell membrane. Lysosomes carry hydrolases that degrade nucleotides, proteins, lipids and phospholipids; they also remove carbohydrate, sulphate, or phosphate groups from molecules. Lysosomes store iron, either as soluble ferritin or as products of ferritin degradation, such as haemosiderin. Abnormalities associated with lysosomal function cause a variety of storage disorders such as Tay–Sachs disease [9].

Peroxisomes are small granules arranged in clusters around the smooth ER and glycogen stores. They contain about 50 enzymes, some of which are used in respiration, purine catabolism and alcohol metabolism. They are responsible for about 20% of the oxygen consumption in the liver via a respiratory pathway that produces heat rather than ATP as its product. They differ from lysosomes in that they are not formed from outgrowths of the Golgi apparatus but are self-replicating, rather like mitochondria. They also play an important role in the metabolism of fatty acids as well as cholesterol and bile acid synthesis.

Non-parenchymal cells of the liver

Stellate cells and myofibroblasts

Hepatic stellate cells (HSC) are star-shaped cells with long cytoplasmic extrusions. They were first described over 150 years ago by von Kupffer, but for many years their function remained a mystery. They are found in the space of Disse adjacent to the overlying endothelium and hepatocytes, and in the normal liver they represent 5–8% of all liver cells. Under resting conditions HSC store retinoids in numerous vitamin A-rich lipid droplets and are thought to regulate sinusoidal blood flow via contractile intracellular filaments. HSC are the principal cells involved in liver fibrosis, remodelling extracellular matrix and synthesising scar tissue in response to liver injury.

Extracellular matrix and liver fibrosis

In every tissue of the body cells are cemented into place by a variety of proteins and proteoglycans which constitute the extracellular matrix (ECM). This protein mat provides a secure foundation for the cells, but its components also have effects on cell function and differentiation. Cellular attachment is mediated by a family of matrix receptors found on the cell surface called integrins. Integrins secure the cell to the matrix, and determine cell shape, migration and spread.

The ECM is produced mainly by hepatic stellate cells and liver fibroblasts, with a contribution from local hepatocytes. It is significantly altered following tissue injury, as local fibroblasts replace the existing matrix with the type 1 collagen that makes up the bulk of fibrotic (scar) tissue in cirrhosis. In chronic liver disease healthy tissue is replaced by tightly packed collagen fibres which form the septal bands that typify fibrosis. Over time the liver scarring becomes so extensive that little healthy tissue remains, resulting in the pathological condition of cirrhosis. It is important to note that fibrosis is a potentially reversible condition, as the liver possesses mechanisms to remove scar tissue, but established cirrhosis represents a stage of scarring so advanced that the liver is unlikely to be able to make a full recovery.

Endothelial cells

The liver contains two forms of endothelium: conventional vascular endothelium, which is mainly localised around the portal tracts and within large vessels, and a specialised endothelium found within the sinusoids. Sinusoidal endothelial cells (SEC) possess unique phenotypic and structural properties that differentiate them from normal capillary vessels, in particular the presence of pores or fenestrations within the cells and the lack of a basement membrane. This permits the free exchange of macromolecules between the sinusoidal lumen and the space of Disse. SEC perform a variety of functions while acting as a barrier between the blood and liver tissue. Endothelial cells can promote recruitment of inflammatory cells from the blood into liver tissue by expression of adhesion molecules on the sinusoidal surface [10]. Under inflammatory conditions these adhesion molecules increase in number and act like 'biological Velcro', causing white blood cells to stick to the endothelium and enter the liver tissue.

Kupffer cells and liver lymphocytes

Kupffer cells are liver macrophages and constitute almost 90% of the total number of tissue macrophages within the body. These phagocytic cells are found in the lumen of the sinusoid and play an important role in immune 'policing', organising the immune response to bacteria and antigens travelling through the portal vein. Macrophages become activated by components of bacterial cell walls as well as by cytokines such as interferon-γ secreted by helper T cells. Once activated, Kupffer cells phagocytose foreign bodies and present antigen to local T cells, which in turn activate the adaptive immune response.

The surface of a Kupffer cell is coated with a variety of receptors for certain classes of antibody. If a foreign body (e.g. a bacterium) is coated with the appropriate antibody then this binds to the complimentary receptor on the Kupffer cell, triggering rapid phagocytosis and destruction of the foreign antigen. Some of this internally digested antigen is then expressed on the membrane, allowing Kupffer cells to activate local T cells. Following activation Kupffer cells secrete a number of important inflammatory cytokines that attract proinflammatory cells to the liver and release interferon-γ, which provides antiviral protection for local cells.

The liver contains large numbers of lymphocytes, which increase in number following tissue injury in response to cytokines and chemokines released by inflamed tissue. Most of the T cells within the liver are mature lymphocytes that have already been programmed to respond to antigen. This large resident population of mature lymphocytes acts as a form of immunological memory.

Unlike blood lymphocytes, there are roughly equivalent numbers of CD4 and CD8 T cells within the liver, as well as large numbers of natural killer (NK) cells, a specialised immune cell that provides a first line of defence, particularly against viral infection.

Cholangiocytes

Cholangiocytes are epithelial cells that line the intrahepatic and extrahepatic biliary tree. Despite being predominantly cuboidal in the smaller interlobular bile ducts, in the intrahepatic and extrahepatic bile ducts they develop into larger specialised columnar cells. They absorb water, and modify bile by secreting bicarbonate and other substances under the influence of hormones and cholinergic innervation. Expression of mitochondrial autoantigens in cholangiocytes and the diversity of biliary epithelia at different sites are thought to explain why diseases such as primary biliary sclerosis and primary sclerosing cholangitis occur at different sites in the biliary tree.

Biliary tree and gallbladder

Bile is produced by hepatocytes from several essential components, including water, bile acids, cholesterol, phospholipids and bilirubin. Most of these substances are absorbed in the distal ileum and delivered to the hepatocyte via the portal vein. The liver excretes approximately 500–600 mL of bile each day, most of which is stored in the gallbladder. Bile acids have an important function in emulsifying lipids in the digestive tract, which improves digestion by pancreatic lipases.

The biliary tree begins with tiny channels (canaliculi) that form between the walls of adjacent hepatocytes. The canaliculi are sealed by tight junctions in the cell wall, which allows the hepatocyte to actively transport components of bile into the canalicular lumen and protects the hepatocyte from its concentrated contents. These canaliculi form a complicated network of tiny passages that run between adjacent hepatocytes towards the portal tract. Bile flows within them towards the portal triad in the opposite direction to the blood flow. At the margin of the lobule the canaliculi drain into bile ductules and merge within the portal tract to form the interlobular bile ducts. As these bile ducts continue to unite they increase in size from approximately 20 μm to 100 μm in diameter to form large segmental bile ducts lined by a specialised columnar epithelium. These segmental ducts conjoin to form the right and left intrahepatic ducts, which as they leave the hilum of the liver unite to form the common hepatic duct.

Outside the liver the common hepatic duct is joined by the cystic duct of the gallbladder and becomes the common bile duct (CBD). The extrahepatic and intrahepatic ducts are supplied with blood by a fine network of tiny arterial branches that originate from the hepatic and gastroduodenal arteries. As it has no other blood supply, the biliary tree is particularly susceptible to ischaemic injury, such as hepatic artery thrombosis or injury to the biliary plexus during laparoscopic surgery. This can result in extrahepatic and complex hilar and perihilar ischaemic strictures of the biliary tree.

As it approaches the duodenum the CBD lies to the right of the hepatic artery and anterior to the portal vein. It passes underneath the first part of the duodenum through a groove in the head of the pancreas and enters the second part of the duodenum, running through the posteromedial portion of the duodenal wall for a short distance, before exiting through the ampulla of Vater.

In the majority of people the pancreatic duct and CBD join within the ampulla to form a common channel with a single opening into the duodenum. The ampulla can be cannulated during procedures such as endoscopic retrograde cholangiopancreatography (ERCP) to obtain X-ray images of the biliary and pancreatic ducts, and it also provides a means of treating obstructive cases of jaundice, such as pancreatic cancer or gallstones (Figure 1.8).

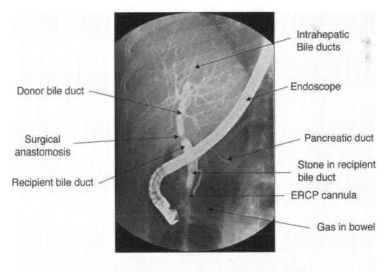

ERCP image of bile ducts following liver transplantation

Figure 1.8 ERCP illustrating bile tract anatomy.

The gallbladder is a hollow organ attached to the lower surface of the liver. It stores 30–50 mL of bile and drains into the common hepatic duct through the cystic duct. The main function of the gallbladder is to store bile and concentrate it even further by absorbing water. This process is mediated by specialised epithelial cells which line the walls of the gallbladder and contain active sodium transport pumps that allow water to be reabsorbed from the lumen against the concentration gradient. This hyperconcentrated bile is then secreted into the bowel through the ampulla by the contraction of the smooth muscle lining in response to the hormone cholecystokinin, which is secreted by the epithelial cells of the small intestine in response to intraluminal fat.

Key points

- The liver is the largest solid organ in the human body and is responsible for many of the vital functions that maintain the health of an individual.
- The liver receives its blood supply from the portal vein, which drains the capillary bed of the digestive tract, and the hepatic artery.
- Blood is drained from the liver via three large hepatic veins, which ultimately drain into the IVC.
- The liver can be divided into eight segments, which are determined by the blood supply from the portal vein.
- The functional unit of the liver is the acinus.
- Hepatocytes constitute approximately 80% of all liver cells, and are the chief functional cell of the liver. They perform various roles, including the metabolism of drugs, protein synthesis, secretion of clotting factors, and the storage of sugar in the form of glycogen.
- Bile is produced by hepatocytes from several components, including bilirubin and bile acids; it is concentrated and stored in the gallbladder.
- Bile is secreted into the bowel when required, where it emulsifies lipids.

Guided further reading

Baynes JW, Dominiczak MH (eds) (2005) *Medical Biochemistry, 2nd edn*. London: CV Mosby.
An introduction to clinical biochemistry.

Kierzenbaum AL (ed) (2002) *Histology and Cell Biology. An Introduction to Pathology*. London: CV Mosby.
An introduction to liver histology.

O'Grady J, Lake RP, Howdle PD (eds) (2000) *Comprehensive Clinical Hepatology.* London: CV Mosby.
A good up-to-date description of liver anatomy and function.

Sadler, TW (ed) (1990) *Langmans Medical Embryology.* Baltimore: Williams & Wilkins, 237–259.
A well-written guide to human embryology and fetal liver anatomy.

References

1. Baron MH. Embryonic origins of mammalian hematopoiesis. *Exp Hematol* 2003; 31: 1160–1169.
2. Deshpande RR, Heaton ND, Rela M. Surgical anatomy of segmental liver transplantation. *Br J Surg* 2002; 89: 1078–1088.
3. Baerg J, Zuppan C, Klooster M. Biliary atresia – a fifteen-year review of clinical and pathologic factors associated with liver transplantation. *J Pediatr Surg* 2004; 39: 800–803.
4. Couinaud C. Liver anatomy: portal (and suprahepatic) or biliary segmentation. *Dig Surg* 1999; 16: 459–467.
5. Thurman RG, Kauffman FC. Sublobular compartmentation of pharmacologic events (SCOPE): metabolic fluxes in periportal and pericentral regions of the liver lobule. *Hepatology* 1985; 5: 144–151.
6. Szczesna-Skorupa E, Chen CD, Liu H, Kemper B. Gene expression changes associated with the endoplasmic reticulum stress response induced by microsomal cytochrome p450 overproduction. *J Biol Chem* 2004; 279: 13953–13961.
7. Wojcik E, Dvorak C, Chianale J, Traber PG, Keren D, Gumucio JJ. Demonstration by in situ hybridization of the zonal modulation of rat liver cytochrome P-450b and P-450e gene expression after phenobarbital. *J Clin Invest* 1988; 82: 658–666.
8. Lieber CS. The discovery of the microsomal ethanol oxidizing system and its physiologic and pathologic role. *Drug Metab Rev* 2004; 36: 511–529.
9. Vellodi A. Lysosomal storage disorders. *Br J Haematol* 2005; 128: 413–431.
10. Lalor PF, Shields P, Grant A, Adams DH. Recruitment of lymphocytes to the human liver. *Immunol Cell Biol* 2002; 80: 52–64.

2

Functions of the liver

Sheetal (Tina) Vaghjiani

Objectives

To outline the liver's role in the following processes:

- Protein handling
- Carbohydrate handling
- Lipid handling
- Bile and bilirubin handling
- Hormone inactivation
- Drug metabolism
- Immunological function

Introduction

In the days of Babylonia the priest–physician would examine minutely the liver of sacrificial animals for signs of import from the gods. The liver was chosen because it contains the most blood; as life and blood were deemed synonymous, the liver was considered the seat of the soul. Throughout much of recorded history there was a belief that the liver was at the centre of things mainly because of the wealth of functions that are apportioned to it.

The liver plays many crucial roles in metabolism and elimination. These functions are facilitated by its anatomy and location, and its generous dual blood supply (as covered in Chapter 1). The liver is composed of a variety of cells, each contributing to overall function, which can be generally described as the regulation of the concentration of solutes in blood that affect the functions of all the other organs of the body. This regulation is achieved by the uptake, metabolism, biotransformation, storage and secretion of endogenous and exogenous solutes and by *de novo* synthesis and secretion.

It is important to gain an understanding of the normal physiology and metabolic pathways of the healthy liver in order to interpret those biochemical changes that occur in the various hepatic pathologies.

Among other things, the liver is responsible for the metabolism of carbohydrate, lipid and protein; these processes are all interlinked, and Figure 2.1 outlines their relationships. The biochemical pathways involved in the metabolism of each of these macronutrients will be dealt with in turn.

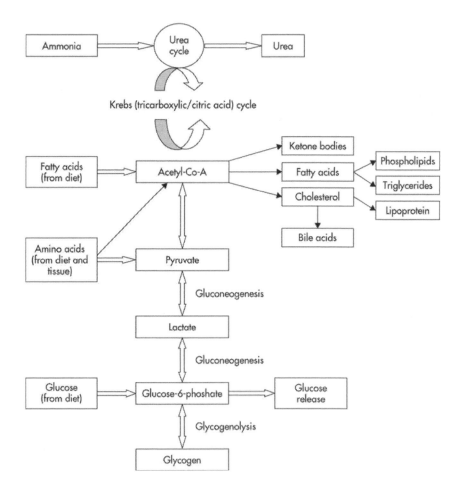

Figure 2.1 Interaction between carbohydrate, lipid and protein metabolism.

Protein handling

Protein synthesis

The liver plays a central role in the synthesis of nearly all circulating proteins. Plasma contains 60–80 g/L of protein and this is turned over at a rate of approximately 250 g/day. A variety of proteins are constructed in the liver using amino acids (Aa) as their basic building blocks. Amino acids are categorised as 'essential' and 'non-essential', the former being a requirement of dietary intake as they cannot be constructed *in vivo*, whereas the latter can be synthesised hepatically. The essential amino acids are further categorised as branched-chain amino acids (BCAA; leucine, valine, isoleucine) or aromatic amino acids (AAA; phenylalanine, tyrosine, methionine) according to their structure. Table 2.1 lists some of the important circulating proteins which are synthesised by the liver, together with their role in healthy subjects and the consequences of liver disease on these systems.

Clotting factors

The liver is the sole site of synthesis of all the clotting factors of the coagulation cascade, apart from Factor VIII, which is largely synthesised by the vascular endothelium. In addition, the liver produces many of the proteins involved in fibrinolysis, such as plasminogen. Figure 2.2 is a diagram of the blood coagulation cascade, which indicates the roles of the clotting factors produced by the liver.

The coagulation cascade is a series of linked biochemical reactions that result in the formation of a durable fibrin clot. Two distinct, but closely linked: interacting pathways are depicted when describing coagulation, the intrinsic and the extrinsic pathways. These pathways have different modes of activation: the intrinsic pathway is activated when blood comes into contact with subendothelial connective tissues as a result of tissue damage, whereas the extrinsic pathway is initiated by the presence of tissue factor, released in response to injury. The intrinsic and extrinsic pathways are measured by the activated partial thromboplastin time (APTT) and prothrombin time (PT), respectively, and these are a good measure of the liver's synthetic function. The key features of this cascade are: (a) activation of Factor X to Factor Xa, where the intrinsic and the extrinsic pathways converge to initiate the 'final common pathway' of coagulation; (b) activation of prothrombin to form thrombin; and (c) formation of the fibrin clot.

Table 2.1 Role of circulating proteins in healthy subjects and those with liver disease

Protein	Role in healthy subjects	In liver disease	Comments
Albumin*	Maintains plasma oncotic pressure. Transports fat-soluble substances, e.g. bilirubin, drugs	Reduced levels Low levels cause ascites and increase free plasma concentration of albumin-bound drugs, e.g. oestradiol, phenytoin	Albumin is a useful clinical indicator of the liver's *synthetic* function. The liver produces and exports up to 12 g of albumin per day. Low levels are also seen in malnutrition, hypercatabolism and nephrotic syndrome. Half-life of 20 days, therefore indicator of chronic liver disease
Clotting factors (I* [Fibrinogen], II [prothrombin], V, VII, IX, X) (see below for clotting cascade)	Individual components of the clotting cascade whose function is dependent and synergistic upon all other clotting factors	There is a reduced production of clotting factors in patients with acute liver failure or cirrhosis (due to reduced synthesis) and in those with deranged lipid absorption (due to decreased vitamin K absorption), which produces an antithrombotic bleeding state and an increased tendency to bruise/bleed	Prothrombin time (PT) and the International Normalised Ratio (INR) are useful indicators of the liver's synthetic function. Vitamin K is required for the production of factors II, VII, IX, and X
α-fetoprotein	Present in the plasma of human foetuses and disappears a few weeks after birth, having no normal role in a healthy adult	Very high levels may indicate primary liver cancer. Rising values in patients with chronic hepatitis are an indicator of the development of hepatocellular carcinoma	α-fetoprotein is normally produced in the foetal liver and yolk sac. It is also used for the second trimester screening of Down's syndrome in pregnancy, where its levels are low. High levels are found in some solid tumours
Caeruloplasmin*	Copper-incorporating α glycoprotein; true function remains unclear but acts as a copper donor and oxidative enzyme	Low caeruloplasmin levels may be seen in cirrhosis (especially primary biliary cirrhosis) as caeruloplasmin is excreted hepatically	Levels increased in infection, injury or inflammation. Low levels are found in Wilson's disease, which is an autosomal recessive disorder of copper metabolism; it results in copper deposition in the liver, basal ganglia and eyes, and culminates in cirrhosis and neurological impairment

Table 2.1 Continued

Protein	Role in healthy subjects	In liver disease	Comments
Transferrin	A high-affinity serum iron transport protein	Transferrin is synthesised in the liver and its levels are diminished in cirrhosis	Iron overload i.e haemochromatosis/haemosiderosis may lead to cirrhosis. A transferrin saturation >55% in males (and postmenopausal women) or >50% in premenopausal women requires investigation to exclude a diagnosis of hereditary haemochromatosis
α_1-antitrypsin*	A serine protease inhibitor synthesised by the liver to limit the plasma circulation of important proteases	α_1-antitrypsin is synthesised in the liver and its levels are diminished in cirrhosis	α_1-antitrypsin deficiency is an inherited autosomal recessive disease. It is characterised by panacinar emphysema of the lungs, and hepatitis in the young, progressing in some to cirrhosis, and culminating in hepatocellular carcinoma in 2–3%
Complement components	Host defence against infectious and inflammatory processes	Complement C3, C5a, B, D, I and P levels are all reduced in hepatitis and cirrhosis	There are 16 components of the complement system, which is divided into the classic and alternative pathways
Haptoglobin	A haemoglobin-binding α_2-globulin that targets aged haemoglobin particles for removal by the liver	Haptoglobin is synthesised in the liver and its levels are diminished in cirrhosis	Haptoglobin levels are raised with inflammatory and infective processes. Serum haptoglobin is used to detect haemolytic anaemia. Other drugs may alter the plasma concentration of haptoglobins, e.g. isoniazid lowers haptoglobin levels

* Indicates acute-phase proteins.

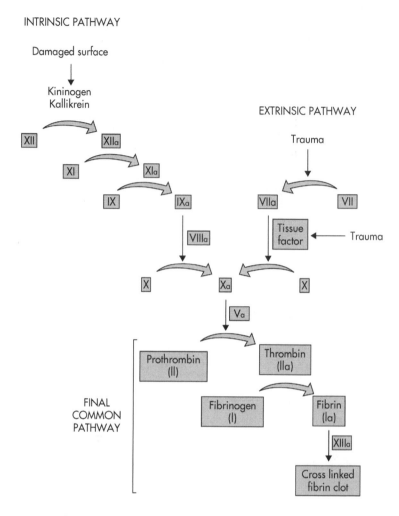

Figure 2.2   The clotting cascade.

Metabolism and degradation

Although the liver is crucial in protein synthesis, it is of equal importance in amino acid metabolism and degradation. This is evidenced by
the high daily turnover of amino acids, and the high proportion of
amino acids that are recycled and reconstituted into new protein
molecules. Over 30 g of protein are irreversibly catabolised (and hence
lost) daily. The nitrogen released from the complete catabolism of
amino acids can be removed by a variety of routes, but the principal

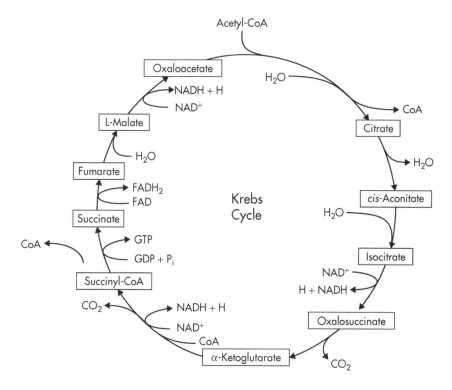

Figure 2.3   The Krebs–citric acid cycle.

pathway is urea synthesis and excretion via the Krebs–Henseleit urea cycle, discussed below.

The portal venous system carries blood from the gastrointestinal tract (GIT) to the liver. This blood carries any nutrients, drugs or toxins that have been absorbed via the enteral route. The liver's handling of drugs and toxins is discussed later in this chapter.

The liver is responsible for modifying blood protein and Aa composition, which it performs by a series of enzymatic process including transamination, deamination and reamination. The essential aromatic amino acids are degraded in the liver, whereas the branched-chain amino acids are passed to the periphery, where they are metabolised exclusively by skeletal muscle. Non-essential amino acids may be metabolised hepatically or in skeletal muscle.

Some Aa are transaminated or deaminated to ketoacids, which are then metabolised by many pathways, including the Krebs–citric acid cycle (Figure 2.3). Others are metabolised to ammonia and urea by the Krebs–Henseleit urea cycle (Figure 2.4).

The Krebs–citric acid cycle is the final common pathway for the oxidation of fuel molecules; amino acids, fatty acids and carbohydrates. Most fuel molecules enter the cycle as a breakdown product, acetyl coenzyme A (acetyl CoA), which reacts with oxaloacetate (a four-carbon compound) to produce citrate (a six-carbon compound), which is then converted in a series of enzyme-catalysed steps back to oxalo-acetate. In the process, two molecules of carbon dioxide and four energy-rich molecules are given off, and these latter are the precursors of the energy-rich molecule ATP, which is subsequently formed and which acts as the fuel source for all aerobic organisms.

Catabolism of amino acids in the liver yields high volumes of ammonia. This can be used in the synthesis of other nitrogenous

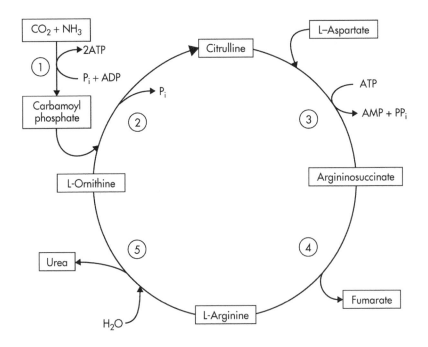

KEY TO ENZYMES (Circled Numbers)

1. Carbamoyl-phosphate synthase
2. Ornithine carbamoyltransferase
3. Argininosuccinate synthase
4. Argininosuccinate lyase
5. Arginase

Figure 2.4 The Krebs–Henseleit urea cycle.

compounds but is highly toxic. Therefore, over 90% of this surplus nitrogen is disposed of by conversion of ammonia to urea via the Krebs–Henseleit urea cycle (Figure 2.4). Although our bodies cannot tolerate high concentrations of urea, it is much less poisonous than ammonia and urea is removed efficiently by the kidneys at a rate of almost 3 g/day. The urea cycle occurs almost exclusively in the liver and consists of a series of metabolic reactions whereby ammonia is converted to urea using cyclically regenerated ornithine as a carrier.

In one turn of the cycle, it:

- Consumes two molecules of ammonia
- Consumes one molecule of carbon dioxide
- Creates one molecule of urea $(NH_2)_2CO$
- Regenerates a molecule of ornithine for another turn.

There are several inherited diseases of the urea cycle caused by mutations in genes encoding one or another of the necessary enzymes. The synthesis of urea in the liver is the major route of removal of ammonia, and any defect in the urea cycle has devastating consequences because there is no alternative pathway for the synthesis of urea, leading to hyperammonaemia. The most common urea cycle disorder is an inherited deficiency of ornithine carbamoyltransferase (OTC), an enzyme needed for the conversion of ornithine to citrulline. The disease is diagnosed on the basis of a hyperammonaemia and hypocitrullinaemia. Other examples of inherited disorders of the urea cycle are carbamoyl phosphate synthetase I and N-acetylglutamate synthase deficiencies. Table 2.2 lists the changes in protein metabolism and degradation seen in liver disease.

Carbohydrate handling

The liver is the principal organ for glucose homoeostasis and maintenance of blood glucose and has an important role in the maintenance of plasma carbohydrate levels. Glucose, which is absorbed from the GIT, is transported to the liver where it is stored as glycogen. Approximately 80 g of glycogen is stored in the liver, and approximately 160 g of glucose per day is needed for normal body functions.

In the 'fed' postprandial state, glucose and fructose are removed from the portal venous blood by the hepatocytes. This allows glucose stores to be formed in the liver as an energy reserve, and also prevents any wide fluctuations in plasma osmolality as a result of a hyperglycaemic state. Within the hepatocyte, glucose is converted

Table 2.2 Changes in protein metabolism and degradation seen in liver disease

Liver injury	Change in levels	Mechanism	Clinical implications
Cirrhosis	Increased plasma concentration of AAA (i.e. reduced metabolism) Normal/reduced plasma concentration of BCAA	These changes are due to imbalances in metabolism of amino acids. BCAAs which are metabolised in muscle are relatively low in concentration as muscle metabolism continues normally. Aromatic amino acids which are metabolised hepatically are present in relatively high concentrations as the deranged liver is unable to perform its usual metabolic functions	Aminoaciduria Change in ratio of AAA/BCAA may be linked to hepatic encephalopathy
	Hyperammonia and low urea levels	Portosystemic shunting of ammonia derived from colonic bacteria. Failure of degradation of Aa to urea	Increased ammonia related to hepatic encephalopathy
Acute liver failure	May be a rise in plasma ammonia and low urea levels	Failure of degradation of Aa to urea	Increased ammonia related to hepatic encephalopathy and cerebral herniation. High ammonia and low urea are diagnostic markers for poor hepatic synthetic function

to glucose-6-phosphate, which is then used for the synthesis of glycogen and/or fatty acids which are subsequently esterified to triglyceride.

In the 'fasting' state the liver is an essential source of energy for other tissues, either by the breakdown of glycogen to glucose (glycogenolysis) or by the production of glucose from lactate, pyruvate, and amino acids from muscle tissue and glycerol from lipolysis of fat stores (gluconeogenesis). During overnight fasting the former is the more important, but its contribution falls rapidly after 24 hours (Table 2.3).

Table 2.3 Changes in carbohydrate handling observed in liver disease

Liver injury	Change in levels	Mechanism	Clinical implications
Cirrhosis	Hyperglycaemia	Portosystemic shunting of insulin and decreased hepatic insulin breakdown leads to inhibition of muscle glucose utilisation and peripheral insulin resistance, leading to elevated glucose levels	Hyperglycaemia, acidosis, osmotic diuresis
Acute liver failure	Hypoglycaemia	Failure of the liver to store glycogen and release glucose due to hepatic dysfunction	Sweating, tachycardia and hypoglycaemic coma may occur

Lipid handling

The liver is central to both lipid and lipoprotein metabolism and homeostasis. There are three major plasma lipids: cholesterol, phospholipids and triglycerides. All are highly insoluble in water.

Cholesterol

Cholesterol is an extremely important biological molecule that modulates the fluidity of animal cell membranes and is the precursor of steroid hormones (such as progesterone, testosterone, oestradiol and cortisol) and bile acids. Cholesterol is either derived from the diet or synthesised *de novo*. Regardless of the source, cholesterol is transported through the circulation in lipoprotein particles, as are cholesterol esters, the cellular storage form of cholesterol. The amount of cholesterol synthesised daily in the liver of a normal person is usually double that obtained from dietary sources. Other sites of cholesterol synthesis include the intestine, and the degree of production is highly responsive to cellular levels of cholesterol. Over 1.2 g of cholesterol is lost in the faeces daily in the form of free sterol or as bile acids.

All 27 carbon atoms of cholesterol are derived from acetyl CoA in a three-stage synthetic process (Figure 2.5):

- Isopentyl pyrophosphate is synthesised from acetyl CoA.

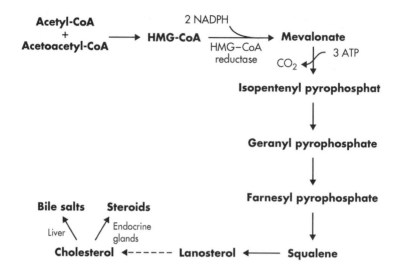

Figure 2.5   Synthesis of cholesterol.

- The six-molecule structure of isopentyl pyrophosphate is condensed to form squalene.
- Squalene cyclises and the tetracyclic product is converted into cholesterol.

The rate-limiting step for cholesterol synthesis is the production of mevalonate from 3-hydroxy-3-methylglutaryl coenzyme A (HMG CoA) by the enzyme HMG-CoA reductase. Cholesterol synthesised in the hepatocyte can be further metabolised by lecithin cholesterol acyl transferase (LCAT) to cholesterol ester, which is packaged into lipoproteins and secreted into the bloodstream. Alternatively, it can be excreted via the biliary system either as a neutral lipid or following conversion to bile acids.

Phospholipids

Phospholipids are a diverse group of compounds; they are fat derivatives in which one fatty acid has been replaced by a negatively charged phosphate group, and one of several nitrogen-containing molecules and an alcohol group. Phospholipids are vital constituents of all cell membranes. The most widespread phospholipid in the plasma is lecithin (phosphatidylcholine), which is synthesised in the liver.

Triglycerides

Triglycerides, along with other lipids and cholesterol, are derived mainly from the diet and transported from the intestine in the form of chylomicrons. Triglycerides are also formed in the liver by esterification of fatty acyl-CoAs with glycerol-3-phosphate. They act as a source of energy and a source of transporting energy from the intestine and liver to the peripheries.

Lipoproteins

Lipoproteins are essential for the transport of lipids from the gut and liver to the tissues, and for lipid metabolism. Lipoproteins are spherical particles with a hydrophobic core, covered by a single layer of amphipathic molecules: phospholipids, cholesterol and one or more apoproteins (of which ten have been isolated; these are produced in the liver). The role of these protein coverings is twofold: they solubilise hydrophobic lipids and contain cell-targeting signals.

These lipids are insoluble in water and are classified on the basis of their ultracentrifugal properties into chylomicrons, very low-density lipoprotein (VLDL), intermediate-density lipoprotein (IDL), low-density lipoprotein (LDL) and high-density lipoprotein (HDL) in order of ascending density. Table 2.4 gives the classification and roles of lipoproteins.

Table 2.4 Classification and roles of lipoproteins

Lipoprotein	Source	Transports
Chylomicron	Gut	Dietary fat
Chylomicron remnants	From chylomicrons	Triglycerides and cholesterol
Very low-density lipoprotein (VLDL)	Liver	Triglycerides and cholesterol
Intermediate-density lipoprotein (IDL)	From VLDL	Cholesterol
Low-density lipoprotein (LDL)	From IDL	Cholesterol
High-density lipoprotein (HDL)	Peripheral tissue	Cholesterol esters

Lipoproteins are metabolised by two main pathways, according to the origin of the lipoprotein particle being handled. The exogenous pathway involves lipids absorbed from the diet, and the endogenous pathway is concerned with synthesised lipid (Figure 2.6).

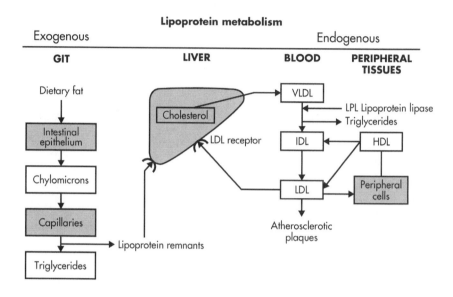

Figure 2.6 Diagram illustrating lipoprotein metabolism.

Exogenous pathway

Chylomicrons are produced from dietary fat by the removal of resynthesised triglycerides from the mucosal cells of the small intestine into the intestinal lumen. These then enter the circulation via the thoracic ducts in the lymphatic system and enter into the subclavian veins, where triglyceride content is reduced by the action of lipoprotein lipases (LPL) on capillary endothelial surfaces in skeletal muscle and fat. The free fatty acids (FFA) from the triglycerides are used by the tissues as an energy source or stored as triglycerides. The chylomicron remnants, stripped of triglyceride and therefore denser, are then taken up by the liver by LDL receptor-mediated endocytosis, thereby delivering cholesterol to the liver.

Endogenous pathway

VLDL particles are assembled in the liver and consist of triglycerides (50–60%) and cholesterol. These particles leave the liver, where the triglyceride load is gradually reduced by the action of lipoprotein lipase to yield free fatty acids for use in the peripheral tissues. The VLDL particle therefore gradually decreases in size as it is transported in the circulation, forming the smaller intermediate-density lipoprotein (IDL) particle.

IDL is partly re-taken up by the hepatocytes for cholesterol recycling. The majority of IDL particles are further stripped of triglycerides, thereby forming LDL, the major carrier of cholesterol.

The LDL particle (10% triglyceride content) is finally taken up into the liver and other tissues by the LDL receptor. The LDL receptor is a six-domain transmembrane protein whose synthesis is under negative feedback regulation, such that when intracellular cholesterol levels are raised, new LDL receptors are not formed, thereby preventing the uptake of further cholesterol from plasma LDL. LDL also inhibits HMG-CoA reductase and hence cholesterol synthesis by negative feedback inhibition. Absence of the LDL receptor leads to hypercholesterolaemia and atherosclerosis, as there is a decrease in the rate at which LDLs are removed from the plasma.

HDL is synthesised and secreted from the liver and gut and aids the removal of cholesterol from peripheral tissues. It opposes the effects of LDL and protects against coronary heart disease. HDL is the substrate for LCAT, which converts the cholesterol in circulating plasma lipoproteins to cholesterol esters, which are then transferred to other lipoprotein particles. This is termed reverse cholesterol transport. Table 2.5 delineates the changes in lipid handling observed in liver disease.

Bile

Bile is a complex fluid containing 95% water, electrolytes and organic molecules, including bile acids/salts, cholesterol, phospholipids and conjugated bilirubin that flows through the biliary tract into the small intestine (Table 2.6).

Bile is produced by the hepatocytes and modified by the cholangiocytes that line the bile ducts. Adults produce approximately 400–800 mL of bile daily. The bile salt-dependent pathway produces approximately 225 mL/day, the bile salt-independent pathway produces approximately 225 mL/day, and cholangiocytes produce a further 150 mL/day.

The bile salt-dependent pathway relies on conjugated bile salts being excreted from the hepatocytes into the hepatic canaliculi via the

Table 2.5 Changes in lipid handling observed in liver disease

Liver injury	Change in levels	Mechanism	Clinical implications
Cholestasis	Increased total and free cholesterol	Four proposed theories: Regurgitation of biliary cholesterol into the circulation Increased hepatic cholesterol synthesis Reduced plasma LCAT Regurgitation of biliary lecithin, effectively shifting cholesterol into plasma	In acute cholestasis, observe 1.5–2 times normal levels of cholesterol In chronic cholestasis, very high levels of cholesterol are noted, especially in primary biliary cirrhosis, postoperative strictures, Alagille's syndrome and progressive familial intrahepatic cholestasis Yellowish epidermal plaques representing cholesterol deposits (xanthelasma, progressing to xanthomas) may be noted Red cell changes observed in cholestasis are due to abnormalities in cholesterol and lipoprotein
	Decrease in cholesterol esters	Reduced plasma LCAT	
	Increase in LDL and lipoprotein X (abnormal)	Lipids providing increased substrate drive. Lipoprotein X is very rich in free cholesterol and lecithin	
Hepatitis	Increase in triglycerides	Accumulation of triglyceride-rich LDL	Hypertriglyceridaemia on venous sampling
	Low cholesterol esters	Reduced formation of LCAT	
Cirrhosis	Total cholesterol is normal or low	Malnutrition, decompensation and hepatic insufficiency	See Chapter 3 on cirrhosis There may be a reduction in the production of sex hormones and cortisol

effect of various transporter proteins (e.g. the bile salt export pump, BSEP and CMOAT/MRP2) and the electrical gradient present across the canaliculi. The conjugated bile acids secreted into the canaliculi exert a large osmotic effect, providing one of the mechanisms responsible for the induction of bile flow. Hence there is good correlation between bile flow and bile salt secretion.

Table 2.6 Composition of hepatic bile

Component	Concentration (mmol/L)
Electrolytes	
Na^+	141–165
K^+	2.7–6.7
Cl^+	77–117
HCO^{3-}	12–55
Ca^{2+}	2.5–6.4
Mg^{2+}	1.5–3.0
Organic anions	
Bile acids	3–45
Bilirubin	1–2
Lipids	
Lecithin	1.4–8.1 g/L
Cholesterol	0.97–3.2 g/L
Proteins	0.02–0.2 g/L
Peptides and amino acids	
Glutathione	3–5
Glutamate	0.8–2.5
Aspartate	0.4–1.1
Glycine	0.6–2.6

The bile salt-independent pathway depends on osmotically active solutes such as glutathione and bicarbonate to generate water flow into the canaliculi. It has been shown that bile flow continues at zero bile salt excretion, i.e. a bile salt-independent process.

Bile acid metabolism and transport

The bile acid molecule is composed of two distinct components: a steroid nucleus and an aliphatic side chain. The two principal primary bile acids (cholanoic acids), cholic acid and chenodeoxycholic acid, are synthesised from cholesterol in the liver. More than 99% of bile acids are conjugated before being secreted by the hepatocytes, allowing them to interact with other molecules within bile, and preventing them from being precipitated in the acidic environment of the small intestine. The most common conjugates formed are those with taurine and glycine owing to the actions of bile acid CoA synthetase and an *N*-acyltransferase, resulting in the formation of bile salts. Other methods of bile acid conjugation, such as glucuronidation and sulphation, occur in very limited quantities in healthy individuals, but this is greatly increased in cholestasis.

The principal functions of bile acids are:

• Maintenance of cholesterol homeostasis. As outlined above, the cholesterol required is either obtained from the diet in the form of chylomicron remnants or is synthesised *de novo*. The synthesis of bile acids from cholesterol and their subsequent excretion in the faeces represent the only significant mechanism for the elimination of excess cholesterol.

• Stimulation of bile flow in the biliary system. The bile salt-dependent pathway, which allows bile flow, is described above.

• Emulsification/absorption of dietary lipid in the intestine. Bile acids are stored in the gallbladder and released into the duodenum when cholecystokinin is released. In the small intestine, bile acids help to solubilise monoglycerides and fatty acids which are formed as the result of the digestion of dietary triglyceride, thereby enhancing the absorption of lipids and the fat-soluble vitamins A, D, E and K.

Some of the bile salts are deconjugated in the small intestine and reabsorbed by passive diffusion. In contrast, conjugated bile salts are actively reabsorbed in the ileum, from where they are transported back to the liver in the portal venous system. Bile salts are finally taken up by the hepatocytes, where deconjugated bile salts undergo reconjugation. These conjugated bile salts, either formed by reconjugation or actively reabsorbed in the ileum, are now ready for secretion into the canaliculi. This efficient recycling is known as the enterohepatic circulation and is estimated to occur up to 15 times in a single day (Figure 2.7). The

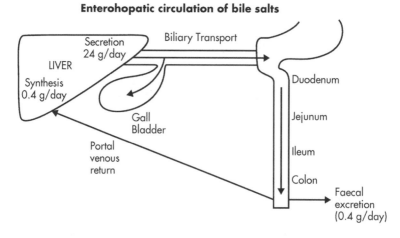

Figure 2.7   Diagram of enterohepatic circulation.

primary bile acids which are not reabsorbed in the ileum undergo biotransformation by colonic bacterial enzymes, cholic acid being converted to deoxycholic acid and chenodeoxycholic acid being converted to lithocholic acid, both by 7α-dehydroxylation. Deoxycholic and lithocholic acid are known as the secondary bile salts. Thus the primary and secondary bile salts make up the four constituents of the bile acid pool. Some deoxycholic acid may be reabsorbed, but only limited quantities of lithocholic acid are recovered. Daily faecal bile acid excretion, composed principally of deoxycholic and lithocholic acid, is in the region of 400 mg/day, and this loss is accounted for by the *de novo* synthesis of new bile acids from cholesterol. Tertiary bile salts, primarily ursodeoxycholic acid, are formed in the liver from secondary bile salts. Tertiary bile salts produce a greater choleresis than do the primary bile acids.

Bilirubin metabolism and transport

Bilirubin is a potentially toxic compound that is an end-product of the breakdown of the porphyrin moiety of haem-containing compounds such as haemoglobin, myoglobin, cytochromes and catalase.

Daily bilirubin production averages 4 mg/kg, and 70–80% is derived from haemoglobin degradation from senescent erythrocytes (which occurs in macrophages in the spleen, liver and bone marrow); a small amount arises from the destruction of developing erythrocytes (ineffective erythropoiesis). The remaining 20–30% of bilirubin production occurs in the liver.

The catabolism of haemoglobin yields haem, which is subsequently converted to bilirubin in a two-step process that takes place in the hepatocyte. First, the microsomal enzyme haem oxygenase cleaves the porphyrin ring of haem, generating biliverdin in an energy-utilising reaction. Following this, biliverdin is converted to bilirubin by the cytosolic enzyme biliverdin reductase. As the liver is the active site for biosynthesis of porphyrin and haem, deficiencies in some enzymes of the porphyrin pathway may lead to insufficient haem production and an increase in porphyrin levels, which causes acute porphyria attacks.

Bilirubin is highly water-insoluble and therefore its elimination from the circulation requires its chemical conversion in the liver to water-soluble conjugates that are normally excreted into the bile. Bilirubin circulates in plasma tightly bound to albumin, and is taken up into the liver by a carrier-mediated process whose competitive inhibition by rifampicin may lead to hyperbilirubinaemia. Bilirubin is then converted to water-soluble monoglucuronides and diglucuronides via conjugation with uridine diphosphate–glucuronic acid, which occurs in the endoplasmic reticulum. This conjugation serves to convert hydrophobic bilirubin into a water-soluble form that can be readily excreted into bile and is under the control of the enzyme bilirubin uridine diphosphate glucuronosyl transferase (bilirubin UGT-1).

Virtually all bilirubin in bile is conjugated, with 80% present in the form of diglucuronides and the remainder as monoglucuronides. Bilirubin is transferred into the duodenum with the normal biliary flow, where it is ultimately eliminated in the stool (and gives stool its colour). Clearly, obstruction of the biliary tree at any level from the canals of Hering to the ampulla of Vater (see Chapter 1) can lead to jaundice. Resorption of conjugated bilirubin by the gallbladder and gut is minimal. However, bilirubin breakdown products may be reabsorbed by the gut, and in particular, conjugated bilirubin may be hydrolysed by bacterial β-glucuronidase in the terminal ileum and colon. The resulting unconjugated bilirubin is converted to urobilinogens in the intestinal lumen, where up to 20% is resorbed by the gut and ultimately excreted in bile and urine (Figure 2.8).

Bilirubin metabolism

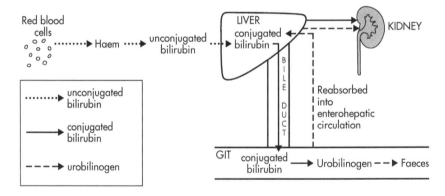

Figure 2.8 Diagram of bilirubin metabolism.

Three inherited disorders of bilirubin metabolism are associated with defects in bilirubin UGT-1 activity: Gilbert's syndrome, and Crigler–Najjar syndrome types I and II. Dubin–Johnson syndrome is due to a defect in the protein pump that extrudes bilirubin from the hepatocyte into the canaliculi. Table 2.7 shows a few of the inherited disorders of bilirubin metabolism and transport. Table 2.8 shows changes in bile handling observed in liver disease.

Hormone inactivation

A large number of hormones are metabolised by the liver, some examples of which are listed below:

- Steroid hormones are conjugated in the liver, e.g. prednisone to prednisolone.
- Cortisol is catabolised to tetrahydrocortisone and subsequently conjugated with glucuronic acid.
- Testosterone is converted to its more potent metabolite, dihydrotestosterone, which is then degraded by the liver and conjugated to 17-oxysteroid, which is excreted in the urine.
- Oestrogens are conjugated for excretion in the urine or bile. In patients with cirrhosis there is a higher proportion of circulating unbound, active oestradiol, a higher concentration of hepatic oestrogen receptors and increased levels of sex hormone-binding globulin, thus reducing the levels of free, active testosterone. This imbalance may cause a shift in physical features towards feminisation, with the appearance of features such as gynaecomastia, loss of secondary sexual hair, female body habitus and impotence. This is particularly true of alcohol-induced cirrhosis.
- Growth hormone.
- Insulin is metabolised within the liver to ensure that its effects are not prolonged, thereby preventing a potentially dangerous hypoglycaemia.
- Aldosterone.
- Thyroxine (T_4) is converted to the biologically active Tri-iodothyronine (T_3) in the liver. The liver has an important role to play in the transport, storage, activation and metabolism of thyroid hormones.

Even in the presence of severe hepatocellular disease, hormone metabolism remains fairly undisturbed. However, hyperinsulinaemia can occur in patients with end-stage cirrhosis, which results in chronic hyperinsulinaemia and then insulin resistance. In cholestasis, the excretion of conjugated hormones such as oestrogen is reduced, resulting in higher blood levels. However, levels of these hormones are difficult to interpret in the presence of liver disease, as feedback mechanisms between plasma levels and hormone secretion prevent chronic rises. In general, hormone levels are a poor guide to hepatic sufficiency, and therefore do not form part of the routine liver function tests because of their unpredictable correlation with hepatic function.

Table 2.7 Inherited disorders of hepatic bilirubin metabolism and transport [1,4]

	Gilbert's syndrome	Type I Crigler–Najjar syndrome	Type II Crigler–Najjar syndrome	Dubin–Johnson syndrome	Rotor's syndrome
Incidence	<10% of population	Extremely rare	Uncommon	Uncommon	Rare
Inheritance	Autosomal recessive	Autosomal recessive	Autosomal recessive	Autosomal recessive	Autosomal recessive
Mechanism	Decreased bilirubin conjugation, as low bilirubin UGT-1 levels	Absent bilirubin conjugation, as no bilirubin UGT-1 levels	Markedly decreased bilirubin conjugation, as minimally active bilirubin UGT-1 levels	Impaired canalicular excretion of conjugated bilirubin	Unknown
Serum bilirubin concentration (μmol/L)	51–68 Virtually all unconjugated	>350 Unconjugated	<350 Virtually all unconjugated	<120 About 50% conjugated	<120 About 50% conjugated

Table 2.8 Changes in bile handling observed in liver disease

Liver injury	Change in levels	Mechanism	Clinical implications
Acute cholestasis	Retention of bile acids	Obstruction of bile flow or bile formation, either extrahepatic (mechanical obstruction) e.g. gallstones or intrahepatic (failure of hepatocytes to generate bile flow) e.g. primary biliary cirrhosis, contraceptive pill	Pruritus Cell necrosis by hepatic bile salts
	Reduction of intestinal bile salts	Reduced biliary excretion of bile salts into the small intestine	Reduced lipid absorption causing steatorrhoea A reduction in vitamin K absorption will cause haematoma, spontaneous bruising and prolonged prothrombin time
	Possible increase in serum conjugated bilirubin	Obstruction of bile flow commonly due to common bile duct stone or pancreatic carcinoma	Extrahepatic cholestasis
Chronic cholestasis	As in acute cholestasis	Failure of bile secretion	Intrahepatic cholestasis Fat malnutrition Reduced levels of fat soluble vitamins will cause:
	Reduction of intestinal bile salts	Reduced secretion of bile acids into the small intestine	A – night blindness, thick skin D – osteomalacia, osteoporosis (multifactoral cause) E – neuromuscular weakness K – clotting abnormalities
	Increase in cholesterol deposition (see above)	Retention of cholesterol normally excreted in the bile	Xanthomas
Cirrhosis	Increased serum bile acid levels	Two hypotheses: 1) The result of haemodynamic alterations, shunts and reduced liver mass 2) Hepatic dysfunction at the cellular level	May lead to pruritus in conditions of bile stasis

Drug metabolism

The liver is a prime site for the metabolism and excretion of many drugs. Most drugs that are presented to the liver undergo hepatic metabolism and are then excreted either in the bile or in the urine.

Lipid-soluble drugs tend to be taken up by the liver and are said to have high first-pass metabolism, which depends on hepatic blood flow. Metabolism of drugs with low hepatic clearance depends on hepatic enzyme capacity.

Once in the liver, drugs undergo a minimum two-stage metabolic process. Phase 1 involves metabolism by cytochrome P450 enzymes, and the second phase includes biotransformation with conjugation of the drug or its metabolites. The drug metabolites produced may be active, e.g. morphine $\rightarrow$ morphine-3-glucuronide and morphine-6-glucuronide; or inactive, e.g. fentanyl. Drug metabolism often leads to the generation of an inactive compound, but reactive and highly toxic intermediates may also be formed. This phenomenon explains the hepatotoxicity of many therapeutic drugs, where the final product is more toxic than the parent compound: this is known as metabolic activation. The pharmacokinetics of an active or intermediary metabolite must be considered when assessing a drug for appropriate use.

Drugs which are highly polar (water soluble) and those drugs that become more polar after conjugation are excreted unchanged in the bile. Those drugs with higher molecular weights (>200 Da) tend to be excreted by the biliary system and those with a lower molecular weight tend to be excreted renally. Alcohol is also metabolised by the liver at a rate of 1 unit/hour. It is broken down by alcohol dehydrogenase and eventually metabolised to acetyl-CoA which then enters the Krebs cycle. See Chapter 5 for a more detailed review of pharmacokinetics and the effect of liver disease.

Immunological function

The liver is intimately involved in systemic and mucosal immunity. It contains the largest pool of mononuclear phagocytes and natural killer cells in the body, and is involved in the transport of secretory IgA into the biliary and upper gastrointestinal tracts. The Kupffer cells provide one of the first lines of defence against gut-derived foreign material, being involved in the uptake and degradation of gut-derived antigens and bacterial products such as endotoxin, as well as the initiation of immunological responses to antigens absorbed from the gut. Liver-associated lymphocytes are a heterogeneous population of cells similar to natural killer cells but with an innate role specific to their location in the liver, chiefly in the response to gut-derived antigens. IgA, the principal immunoglobulin of mucosal immunity, is made within the biliary system and has a vital role in the defence of the biliary and upper GI tracts from the clearance of harmful antigens delivered from the portal circulation.

Summary of liver functions

- Production of plasma proteins.
- Synthesis of clotting factors.
- Regulation of blood levels of amino acids, which form the building blocks of proteins.
- Conversion of poisonous ammonia to urea.
- Conversion of excess glucose into glycogen for storage (this can later be converted back to glucose for energy).
- Synthesis and metabolism of cholesterol, phospholipids, triglycerides and lipoproteins.
- Production of bile, which helps carry away waste and break down fats in the small intestine during digestion. Fats and fat-soluble vitamins A, D, E and K need bile in order to be absorbed.
- Enterohepatic circulation of bile salts.
- Conjugation and excretion of bilirubin.
- Hormone inactivation.
- Metabolism and excretion of drugs and toxins.
- Resisting infection by producing immune factors and removing bacteria from the bloodstream.

This brief summary of the functions of the liver is not intended to replace larger texts on the subject, but to provide a concise account to facilitate an understanding of deranged liver function in the diseased state, with particular relevance to pharmacopathology. Several textbooks of hepatology are recommended for a more comprehensive review of this large topic (see below).

Acknowledgement

With special thanks to Dr Jitinder Paul Singh Saini BSc, MBBS.

Further reading

Berg JM, Tymoczko JL, Stryer L (eds) (2002) *Biochemistry*, 5th edn. New York: WH Freeman and Company.

Kumar P, Clarke M (eds) (2002) *Clinical Medicine*, 5th edn. London: WB Saunders.

MacSween RNM, Burt AD, Portmann BC, Ishak KG, Scheuer PJ, Anthony PP (eds) (2002) *Pathology of the Liver*, 4th edn. London: Churchill Livingstone.

O'Grady JG, Lake JR, Howdle PD (eds) (2006) *Comprehensive Clinical Hepatology*, 2nd edn. London: Mosby.

Sherlock S, Dooley J (eds) (2002) *Diseases of the Liver and Biliary System*, 11th edn. Oxford: Blackwell.

3

Causes of liver disease and dysfunction

Bridget Featherstone

Objectives

- To give an overview of the classification and types of liver disease.
- To give an overview of some of the common conditions that cause liver disease and outline the impact they have on liver function.

Introduction

The liver is a complex organ fulfilling a range of functions and has a remarkable ability for regeneration. It is therefore not surprising that liver disease can manifest in a broad spectrum of conditions, from mild and self-limiting to severe with high mortality. In line with this, the functioning capacity of the diseased liver can extend from normal to severely compromised. The aim of this chapter is to provide an outline of the common causes of liver disease and to describe the types and range of liver dysfunction associated with those diseases.

Classification of liver disease

Liver disease can be classified according to both the pattern of damage seen and the time course over which the damage occurs. The main patterns of damage are initially cholestasis or hepatocellular, both of which can lead to fibrosis, which in turn can lead to cirrhosis. These are not distinct entities and overlap between them is common. In some cases liver disease is self-limiting; however, in others, if left untreated the disease may progress to end-stage liver disease, where the functioning capacity of the liver may be significantly compromised. Liver disease is also classified according to the time course it takes: acute, if the onset of symptoms does not exceed six months, or chronic, if symptoms persist for more than six months.

Cholestasis

Cholestasis is the stagnation of bile along the bile ducts. This disruption of bile flow may be at the level of the intrahepatic biliary ductules, as seen for example in primary biliary cirrhosis, or it may be due to an extrahepatic mechanical obstruction of the bile ducts, as seen for example with cholangitis or gallstones. In either case cholestasis often results in elevated blood levels of substances excreted via the bile and of liver enzymes associated with the biliary tract, notably conjugated bilirubin, alkaline phosphatase, γ-glutamyltranspeptidase, bile acids, and cholesterol. The accumulation of these substances often leads to symptoms such as jaundice, pruritus and xanthelasma. Cholestasis affects liver function and drug handling in two main ways: first, the stagnation of bile flow impairs biliary excretion of certain drugs excreted via this route, for example ceftriaxone; second, as a result of decreased bile excretion, cholestasis reduces the solubility and absorption of fatty substances, for example fat-soluble vitamins, from the gastrointestinal tract. Bile salts themselves are also toxic to the liver, and their accumulation within the liver can damage the hepatocytes, which may lead to fibrosis and cirrhosis.

Hepatocellular disease

Injury to the hepatocytes, for example by hepatotoxins or viruses, will result in hepatocellular damage. This generally manifests itself as fatty infiltration (steatosis), inflammation (hepatitis) or cell death (necrosis). If the assault is mild and remits, the liver will recover and overall liver function will remain normal. Sustained injury causing hepatocyte cell death will, however, ultimately lead to fibrosis and cirrhosis and potentially severe liver dysfunction.

Steatosis

The liver is the principal organ of fat metabolism and, as a result, damage to the hepatocytes can disrupt normal fat metabolism and lead to steatosis: the accumulation of fat within the hepatocytes. Steatosis or fatty liver can be classified into two categories based on the size of the fat droplets deposited within the hepatocyte: microvesicular or

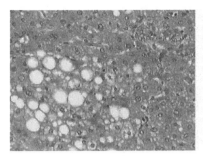

- The appearance of the hepatocytes on the right of this image is normal.
- The cells on the left show a large empty-looking space. This is the position of the fat that has been extracted during the histological processing.

Figure 3.1   Microscopic medium-high-power view of a macrovesicular fatty liver.

macrovesicular. Under a microscope, microvesicular fatty change can be seen as numerous tiny fat vesicles filling the hepatocyte. This may be seen, for example, as a result of drug toxicity with tetracyclines. Microvesicular steatosis is a toxic condition causing hepatocellular failure. Macrovesicular steatosis appears as a few large clear vacuoles in the cytoplasm of hepatocytes which push the nucleus to one side (Figure 3.1). This occurs typically in alcoholic steatosis. Macrovesicular steatosis has less effect on the function of the hepatocyte and liver function tests are usually only minimally abnormal. The accumulation of fat within the hepatocyte may trigger an inflammatory response: this inflammation within the hepatocyte, or hepatitis related to steatosis, is termed steatohepatitis. Continued inflammatory responses further damage hepatocytes, and the liver disease may then progress to fibrosis and cirrhosis.

Hepatitis

Hepatocyte damage or death (necrosis) within the liver evokes an inflammatory reaction that is characterised by the appearance of inflammatory cells together with oedema and congestion around the hepatocytes. This is hepatitis. The inflammation may be acute or chronic. Death of a single or small group of hepatocytes may leave the endoplasmic reticulum intact, in which case cell regeneration will occur and the damage will be completely repaired without liver function being affected. However, if hepatitis is severe and widespread the functioning capacity of the liver may be significantly reduced. With extensive hepatocyte injury the endoplasmic reticulum will become damaged and healing can only occur by the formation of scar tissue, resulting in fibrosis and cirrhosis.

Fibrosis and cirrhosis

In the fibrotic liver active deposition of collagen occurs in response to liver cell injury, resulting in the formation of scar tissue. This fibrosis, or scar tissue, disrupts the blood flow through the liver and obstructs the free passage of substances from the blood to the hepatocytes. Fibrous bands may also form bridges between different areas of the liver. The living cells between these bands attempt to regenerate; however, regeneration is erratic and small nodules are formed that further disturb both the normal liver architecture and the blood flow through the liver. This is the formation of cirrhosis (Figure 3.2). Histologically liver cirrhosis is characterised by widespread nodules in the liver combined with fibrosis. Cirrhosis may further progress in some cases via malignant transformation to hepatocellular carcinoma. The effect of cirrhosis on the functioning capacity of the liver is described below.

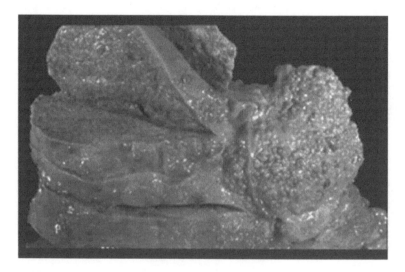

Figure 3.2   Picture of a cirrhotic liver.

Acute versus chronic liver disease

Liver disease is defined as being acute when the history of the onset of symptoms does not exceed six months. The most common causes of acute liver disease in both adults and children are viral hepatitis and drug reactions. Acute hepatitis is usually self-limiting with spontaneous recovery, although in some cases acute liver failure develops and in other cases it may progress to chronic liver disease. Acute liver failure can be defined as hyperacute, acute or subacute, depending on the time from jaundice to encephalopathy [1]. In all classes coagulopathy is present. If encephalopathy occurs within seven days of the onset of jaundice a definition of hyperacute liver failure is given. If encephalopathy occurs within eight to 28 days of jaundice the liver failure is defined as acute. Encephalopathy occurring one to three months after the onset of jaundice is defined as subacute liver failure. In all cases management is based on critical care and liver transplantation, as appropriate. See Table 3.1 for the features of subtypes of acute liver failure.

Liver disease is defined as being chronic when it persists for more than six months. Chronic liver disease develops when permanent structural changes occur within the liver following long-standing cell damage. It usually starts with hepatitis, an inflammation of the hepatocyte that may then progress to fibrosis and then to cirrhosis, as explained above. Initially patients with chronic liver disease will still have enough hepatocyte capacity to perform the functions of the liver: they are described as having 'compensated' liver disease. In the advanced stages of chronic liver disease the remaining capacity of the liver is insufficient for it to carry out its normal functions, metabolism becomes badly affected, and the stage of 'decompensated' chronic liver disease is reached. The disordered anatomy of cirrhosis prevents blood flow through the liver, thereby causing an increased blood pressure within the portal system, leading to portal hypertension. Portal hypertension is a common complication of cirrhosis and is an important factor when considering drug handling in liver disease. The severity of chronic liver

Table 3.1 Features of subtypes of acute liver failure (reproduced with permission from Hospital Pharmacist 2002 p132)

Feature	Hyperacute	Acute	Subacute
Jaundice to encepalopathy (days)	0–7	8–28	29–84
Cerebral oedema	Common	Common	Rare
Renal failure	Early	Late	Late
Ascites	Rare	Rare	Common
Coagulopathy	Marked	Marked	Modest
Prognosis	Moderate	Poor	Poor

disease can be assessed using different models, for example the Child–Pugh classification, which are described in Chapter 4. Liver disease may also be described as 'acute on chronic'. This is when a previously stable patient with chronic liver disease develops a sudden acute clinical complication such as bleeding from oesophageal varices in a cirrhotic patient. The commonest causes of chronic liver disease in adults are alcohol and chronic viral hepatitis. Biliary atresia and α_1-antitrypsin deficiency are the most common causes of chronic liver disease in children. Many other conditions may also lead to chronic liver disease, as described further in this chapter. Management of chronic liver disease is based on treating the underlying condition where possible, treating the symptoms and complications as they arise, and surveying for hepatocellular carcinoma. Transplantation is also a treatment option for certain patients.

Causes of liver disease

Alcoholic liver disease

Alcohol intake is the most important cause of liver cirrhosis in the Western world [2]. Data from the World Health Organization show that the incidence of chronic liver disease and cirrhosis associated with alcohol in the UK is 10.42 per 100 000 people [3]. Interestingly, only around 10–30% of heavy persistent alcohol drinkers will develop liver cirrhosis [2]. The reason why this figure is so low remains unclear. Other factors, such as gender [4,5], genetic makeup [6–8], nutritional status and environmental influences, for example viral infection [9], are likely to play a role.

When taken in small quantities alcohol is metabolised by oxidation, mainly in the liver, to acetylaldehyde and then to acetate by aldehyde dehydrogenase, and then to water, carbon dioxide and fatty acids. When taken regularly in higher quantities a second metabolic pathway, the microsomal ethanol oxidizing system, is also used. This involves the enzyme cytochrome P450 2E1, which increases the metabolism of alcohol to unstable free radicals. By inducing the activity of this enzyme, chronic alcohol consumption increases the metabolism not only of alcohol but also of other drugs metabolised by this route, for example paracetamol. The production of free radicals leads to oxidative stress, altered protein function and the accumulation of fats within the hepatocyte, resulting in hepatitis (hepatocyte inflammation). In some patients this may progress to fibrosis and cirrhosis.

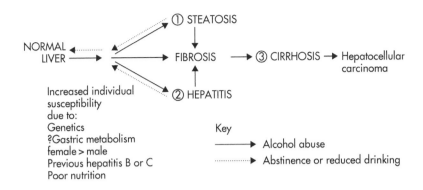

Figure 3.3 Susceptibility to and stages of alcoholic liver disease.

There are three main histological stages of alcoholic liver disease, as highlighted in Figure 3.3: stage 1, steatosis (fatty infiltration of the hepatocyte); stage 2, alcoholic hepatitis; and stage 3, fibrosis and cirrhosis.

Although these stages are pathologically distinct, in practice there is some overlap between them. Macrovesicular steatosis is a predictable histological abnormality that develops in many heavy drinkers. It will reverse within several weeks provided the patient abstains from alcohol, and in general will only have a minimal effect on liver function [10]. Alcoholic hepatitis is characterised by hepatocellular injury with associated inflammation and fibrosis. Alcohol can cause acute and chronic hepatitis, ranging from a mild hepatitis where abnormal liver function tests are the only indicator of disease, to severe liver dysfunction. Severe acute alcoholic hepatitis, with encephalopathy, renal failure, coagulopathy or jaundice, has a poor prognosis. Acute alcoholic hepatitis will usually improve with abstinence from alcohol, although 18% of people will go on to develop cirrhosis despite abstinence [11]. If alcohol misuse continues then inflammation may trigger the formation of fibrosis and ultimately alcoholic cirrhosis. Alcoholic cirrhosis progresses to hepatocellular carcinoma in approximately 5–15% of patients.

Viral infections

Viral hepatitis refers to viral infections that specifically target the liver. There are at least five viruses that cause hepatitis without significant damage to other organs: hepatitis A (HAV), B (HBV), C (HCV), D (HDV) and E (HEV). These viruses may result in an acute infection with hepatitis (A, B, C, D, E) or persistent infection with chronic hepatitis (B, C, D), sometimes leading to cirrhosis and hepatocellular carcinoma. Other viruses that infect and damage other tissues of the body may also cause hepatitis, including Epstein–Barr, cytomegalovirus (CMV), herpes simplex and zoster, Coxsackie A and B, Lassa fever, measles, and the Ebola virus.

Hepatitis A (HAV)

Hepatitis A is the commonest form of infective hepatitis. It is transmitted enterically via the faecal–oral route, and hence is more prevalent in areas of poor sanitary conditions. The incubation period is between 15 and 50 days. In younger patients the disease is usually mild with a very good prognosis, although it may rarely present as acute liver failure. Adults are likely to have more severe disease with large rises of transaminases. Cholestasis is seen commonly in this group, with accompanying jaundice and pruritus. Hepatitis A infection does not progress to chronic liver disease or to carrier status.

Hepatitis B (HBV)

Hepatitis B is highly contagious and is another common cause of infective hepatitis. It is estimated to affect more than two billion people worldwide [12], with a carrier rate of approximately 0.1–0.2% in Western populations and up to 20% in populations in endemic countries in Africa and the Far East. HBV is present in saliva, urine, semen, vaginal fluids and plasma. It is transmitted by contact with infected body secretions, either parenterally, after sexual contact or during birth. The clinical course of hepatitis B depends on the age of the individual when infected. Infants infected by vertical transmission during birth do not usually show signs of disease. However 80–95% of them will develop chronic infection, and around 50% of these will go on to develop liver cirrhosis with or without hepatocellular carcinoma [13]. In adults prodromal symptoms of fever, arthralgia and malaise are commonly seen. These are followed by increases in serum transaminases to between 300 and 800 IU/L, with jaundice following in around half of the cases. Hepatitis B infection is self-limiting in 90–95% of adults, with most patients recovering one to two months after the onset of jaundice. Chronic infection, with viraemia and hepatic inflammation continuing for more than six months, occurs in approximately 5–10% of infected adults. The majority of these run a relatively benign course, although

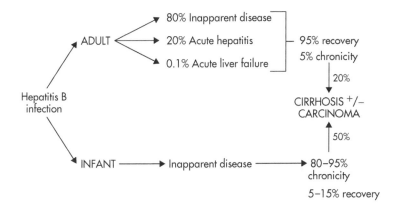

Figure 3.4   The progression of hepatitis B infection.

around 20% will develop cirrhosis over a 5–20-year period and will also run the risk of hepatocellular carcinoma (Figure 3.4). Other factors may affect the course of HBV: for example, those also infected with hepatitis C or D are more likely to develop cirrhosis and hepatocellular carcinoma than those infected with just hepatitis B [14].

Hepatitis D (HDV)

The hepatitis D virus, also known as the Delta virus, is replication defective in humans: it can only replicate in the presence of HBV, and is acquired in the same way. Infection may occur at the same time as the hepatitis B infection (co-infection) or an individual infected with hepatitis B may acquire hepatitis D at a later date (superinfection). The combination of hepatitis B with hepatitis D significantly increases the risk of progression to chronic hepatitis and cirrhosis.

Hepatitis C (HCV)

The hepatitis C virus was defined in 1989. Prior to this, hepatitis following blood transfusion that was not caused by hepatitis A or B was referred to as non-A, non-B hepatitis. HCV is a positive, single-stranded RNA virus of the Flaviviridae family. HCV can be subdivided into groups depending upon the genotype of the virus, which may be important in determining the severity of the disease and the response to treatment. It has been estimated that around 170 million people worldwide are infected with hepatitis C [15]. HCV is primarily transmitted via blood and blood products. The use of unscreened blood transfusions, and re-use of needles and syringes that have not been adequately sterilised, are major transmission routes for HCV. Transmission can also occur sexually, via tattooing, electrolysis, ear piercing, acupuncture, or vertical transmission from mother to foetus. The transmission rate from an HCV-carrier mother to her child is less than 10%, unless the mother is also co-infected with HIV, when transmission rates increase to 19% [16]. Many people with HCV have no obvious risk factor, but have probably been inadvertently exposed to contaminated blood. Up to 85% of people acutely infected with HCV will become chronically infected. Most cases of acute infection are clinically undetectable, although rarely acute liver disease and even liver failure may occur. The natural course of chronic hepatitis C infection varies between individuals: some will have insignificant or minimal liver disease and never develop complications, whereas others will have signs of chronic hepatitis that, if left untreated or if unresponsive to therapy, may develop into cirrhosis. The cirrhosis may progress to end-stage liver disease, in which case the patient will need to be considered for liver transplantation. Individuals with hepatitis C-induced liver cirrhosis are at increased risk of developing hepatocellular carcinoma.

Hepatitis E (HEV)

Individuals infected with HEV show a similar clinical course to those infected with HAV. It is transmitted via the faecal–oral route, with an incubation period of between two and nine weeks. The illness is usually mild, with liver function tests returning to normal within three weeks. It does not progress to chronic liver disease or to carrier status. The main concern of hepatitis E infection is during pregnancy, where the maternal mortality rate is 20% and where miscarriage can occur at any stage. It is not clear why it is more aggressive in this subgroup.

Non-alcoholic fatty liver disease (NAFLD) and non-alcoholic steatohepatitis (NASH)

NAFLD has recently emerged as one of the most common causes of abnormal liver function tests [17]. The overall prevalence of NAFLD in the developed world is estimated to be potentially as high as 20–30% of the population, although the true prevalence remains elusive owing to the lack of a definitive diagnostic test [18]. NAFLD occurs when triglycerides accumulate within the hepatocytes in the absence of heavy drinking, resulting in steatosis. This steatosis may progress to cause hepatocyte inflammation, in which case it is known as non-alcoholic steatohepatitis (NASH). Further progression of disease may occur, resulting in fibrosis and cirrhosis, and in some patients hepatocellular carcinoma. More obese, older and diabetic patients are at greatest risk of developing cirrhosis. NAFLD can be caused by nutritional and endocrine disorders and also by assault to the hepatocytes by chemical compounds, e.g. certain drugs. NAFLD represents the hepatic manifestation of the metabolic syndrome and is related to obesity, insulin resistance, type 2 diabetes, hypertension and hyperlipidaemia. The prevalence of NAFLD is higher in obese than in lean patients, and this difference is associated with the increased prevalence of diabetes in the obese population [19]. Paradoxically, metabolic changes resulting from starvation, excess dieting and protein malnutrition can also lead to fatty infiltration in the hepatocyte and NAFLD.

The initial clinical features of NAFLD are often nondescript. Most patients do not have signs or symptoms of liver disease, although some will report malaise or a feeling of fullness in the right upper quadrant. Hepatomegaly may be present. Laboratory tests characteristically reveal mild elevations of alanine aminotransferase and aspartate aminotransferase.

Initially NAFLD or NASH will have little effect on liver function; however, with progression to fibrosis and cirrhosis the functioning capacity of the liver will decline.

Drugs and toxins

The incidence of drug-induced liver disease appears to be increasing, probably as a result of the increasing number of new drugs being brought onto the market. There have certainly been a number of cases of early drug withdrawal from the market because of drug-induced hepatotoxicity, for example trioglitazone, bromfenac. Over 600 medicinal agents have been associated with causing hepatotoxicity [20]. Certain risk factors may predispose an individual to drug-induced liver disease, as indicated in Table 3.2. Pre-existing liver dysfunction does not generally increase the risk of developing drug-induced liver disease, although exceptions to this have been seen with methotrexate, other cytotoxic agents, aspirin and sodium valproate.

As with any adverse drug reaction, drug-induced liver disease can be described as intrinsic or idiosyncratic. Intrinsic reactions occur when

Table 3.2 Examples of host factors that may predispose to drug hepatotoxicity

Host factor	Comments and drug examples
Gender	
Female	Hepatic drug reactions are more common in females, the reasons for which are unknown. For example, reactions to halothane, isoniazid and nitrofurantoin are more common in females
Male	Reactions to co-amoxiclav are more common in males
Age	
Older	The elderly are at increased risk of adverse drug reactions in general due to altered pharmacokinetics and polypharmacy. For example, reactions to halothane, chlorpromazine, flucloxacillin and co-amoxiclav are more common in elderly patients
Younger	Hepatic drug reactions are rare in children, but may occur with certain drugs such as aspirin and sodium valproate
Pre-existing liver disease	In general patients with pre-existing liver disease are not at increased risk of drug-induced hepatotoxicity; exceptions to this include methotrexate and sodium valproate
Genetics	Genetic differences in drug metabolising enzymes may predispose certain patients to hepatotoxicity. For example, the black and Hispanic population may be more prone to isoniazid toxicity Genetics may play a role in diclofenac hepatotoxicity
Concurrent diseases	
Obesity	Halothane
Diabetes mellitus	Methotrexate
Renal failure	Allopurinol, IV tetracycline
Malnutrition	Paracetamol
HIV positive with hepatitis C or B co-infection	Ibuprofen, ritonauir
HIV positive	Dapsone, cotrimoxazole
Polypharmacy	For example, NSAIDs if used with other hepatotoxic drugs increase the risk of hepatotoxicity. Isoniazid with rifampicin or pyrazinamide

the drug or metabolite causes liver injury in a predictable, reproducible and dose-dependent manner. Idiosyncratic reactions are not predictable or reproducible and occur at a low incidence in individuals exposed to the drug. Idiosyncratic reactions may result from a metabolic idiosyncrasy or from an immunoallergic reaction (Table 3.3).

Drugs can induce almost all forms of acute or chronic liver disease, resulting in a range of damage from minor changes to massive hepatic necrosis. In most instances, withdrawal of the drug will lead to resolution of the liver damage. It is therefore important always to consider the possible contribution of drugs in a patient with any type of liver damage. Table 3.4 lists some drugs implicated and it can be seen from this that individual drugs may cause different types of liver disease.

Inherited and metabolic disorders

A wide range of conditions fall into this group. They can be roughly categorised further into those causing cholestatic disease, chronic liver disease, acute liver failure/metabolic crisis, storage disorders, disorders of bilirubin metabolism. Table 3.5 summarises the types of liver disease that fall into each group.

Alagille's syndrome

This is an autosomal dominant hereditary disorder characterised by a progressive loss of the bile ducts within the liver and narrowing of the bile ducts outside the liver. It is also associated with congenital heart disease, and in particular pulmonary stenosis. Symptoms are related to chronic cholestasis and include jaundice, pruritus, pale loose stools and poor growth within the first three months of life. The majority of children have a benign course and many cases go undetected; however, there is an overall mortality of 20–30% due to progressive liver disease with the development of cirrhosis, cardiac disease or intercurrent infection.

α_1-antitrypsin deficiency (α_1-ATD)

α_1-Antitrypsin is a protein that protects tissues from attack by digestive enzymes, such as trypsin. A deficiency in α_1-antitrypsin causes emphysematous lung disease in adults or liver disease usually in the neonatal period, although liver disease may occur in late childhood and adults. It is the most common genetic cause of liver disease in children. It presents

Table 3.3 Intrinsic vs idiosyncratic hepatotoxic reactions

	Dose dependent	Predictable	Latency	Type of injury and clinical features	Examples
Idiosyncratic toxicity Metabolic abnormality	No	No	Weeks–months	Any Increased liver enzymes, hepatitis, jaundice	Diclofenac Ketoconazole
Idiosyncratic toxicity Immunoallergic reaction	No	No	1–5 weeks	Any Fever, rash, eosinophilia, arthralgias, hepatitis	Halothane Carbamazepine
Intrinsic toxicity Direct toxicity	Yes	Yes	Hours	Usually necrosis Acute liver failure	Paracetamol

Table 3.4 Examples of types of drug-induced liver injury and associated drugs

Pattern of damage	Associated drugs (examples)
Cholestasis	Oral contraceptives, ciclosporin, tamoxifen, warfarin, azathioprine, carbimazole
Acute hepatocellular failure	Allopurinol, aspirin, cocaine, cyclophosphamide, dantrolene, halothane, isoniazid, ecstasy, methyldopa, NSAIDs
Steatosis	Amiodarone, steroids, tetracycline, sodium valproate, tamoxifen, TPN, didanosine
Hepatitis – acute	Dantrolene, isoniazid, phenytoin
Hepatitis – chronic active	Methyldopa, nitrofurantoin, isoniazid
Hepatitis with cholestasis	Chlorpromazine, tricyclics, erythromycin, flucloxacillin, co-amoxiclav, ACE inhibitors, phenytoin, NSAIDs, ranitidine, propafenone, ketoconazole, azathioprine, gold salts, penicillamine
Hepatitis – granulomatous	Phenytoin, allopurinol, carbamazepine, sulphonamides, sulphonylureas
Fibrosis and cirrhosis	Methotrexate, methyldopa, vitamin A
Vascular disorders	
Budd–Chiari syndrome	Oral contraceptives
Veno-occlusive disease	Azathioprine, dactinomycin, dacarbazine, cyclophosphamide
Benign hepatic adenomas	Oral contraceptives

with conjugated hyperbilirubinaemia, hepatomegaly and poor feeding. The extent of liver disease in patients with α_1-ATD can be divided into four different phenotypic groups: 25% have entirely normal liver function; 25% have mild hepatitis but no progression of their liver disease; 25% have jaundice that resolves, but who continue to have hepatomegaly and eventually develop cirrhosis, which ultimately decompensates; and 25% have prolonged cholestasis which progresses to end-stage liver disease and death (or liver transplantation) within a year.

Wilson's disease

Wilson's disease is an inherited disorder of copper metabolism. Copper accumulates initially in the liver and then in the nervous system, leading to severe liver and neurological disease. The retention of copper begins at birth, but it may take decades before the liver is sufficiently damaged

Table 3.5 Examples of inherited and metabolic disorders resulting in liver disease

Type of disorder	Disease
Cholestatic	Alagille's syndrome Progressive familial intrahepatic cholestasis
Chronic	α_1-antitrypsin deficiency Wilson's disease Tyrosinaemia Haemochromatosis Cystic fibrosis
Acute liver failure/metabolic crisis	Galactosaemia Neonatal haemochromatosis Tyrosinaemia Urea cycle disorders Fatty acid oxidation defects
Storage disorders	Glycogen storage diseases Gaucher's disease Wolman's disease
Disorders of bilirubin metabolism	Gilbert's syndrome Dubin–Johnson syndrome Crigler–Najjar syndrome

for symptoms of liver disease to occur. It can present as chronic hepatitis, asymptomatic cirrhosis or acute liver failure, or as cognitive impairment with neuropsychiatric symptoms.

Tyrosinaemia type 1

Tyrosinaemia type 1 is a genetic inborn error of metabolism associated with severe liver disease in infancy. The enzyme responsible for the final step in the degradation of tyrosine is missing, resulting in the formation of highly reactive metabolites (maleyl- and fumaryl-acetoacetate) which are mutagenic to liver cells. Children may present early, in the first month of life, with acute liver failure, or later in childhood with chronic liver disease (failure to thrive, coagulopathy and hepatosplenomegaly) and neurological symptoms. Drug therapy with nitisinone prevents all tyrosine degradation and can rapidly reverse acute liver failure, but there is a significant risk of hepatocellular carcinoma developing in both groups even with treatment, and liver transplantation is ultimately likely to be required.

Haemochromatosis

Haemochromatosis is a recessive genetic condition causing an error in metabolism that results in the body absorbing and storing too much iron. Many individuals with this condition will have no symptoms and liver function will not be affected. However, iron stored in the liver can cause hepatocyte damage that may progress from hepatitis to liver cirrhosis and end-stage liver disease. In the neonatal period it presents as acute liver failure in the first 24 hours of life, with most infants dying within the first month.

Cystic fibrosis

Cystic fibrosis (CF) is a common hereditary disorder of ion transport. Increasing numbers of CF patients are surviving beyond childhood, resulting in an increase in the number of patients with manifestations of hepatobiliary involvement. About one-third of CF patients have abnormal liver function tests, with fatty infiltration occurring in about 70% of older patients [21]. Inspissated secretions within the biliary tree result in obstruction and periductular inflammation that eventually progresses to biliary fibrosis and then multilobular cirrhosis. Hepatomegaly is common. Cholecystitis (inflammation of the gallbladder) is also common, and gallstones occur increasingly with age.

Galactosaemia

Galactosaemia is a rare disease caused by elevated levels of galactose in the blood resulting from a deficiency of the liver enzyme galactose-1-phosphate uridyl transferase (GAL-1-PUT), required to break it down. The disease usually appears in the first few days of life following the introduction of milk. It may present acutely with hypoglycaemia, encephalopathy and liver failure, or more gradually with vomiting, hepatomegaly and jaundice. Removal of galactose and lactose from the diet usually results in a rapid improvement in liver function unless liver failure or cirrhosis has already developed. If dietary measures are not adhered to then fibrosis and cirrhosis may occur.

Glycogen storage diseases (GSD)

This is a group of recessive genetic disorders resulting in defects in glycogen synthesis or breakdown, with each type (and there are several) being caused by a specific enzyme deficiency. This deficiency results in a deranged homoeostasis of glucose and glycogen, leading to an accumulation of hepatotoxic metabolites. Children often present with hepatomegaly, hypoglycaemia and growth failure, and other symptoms depending on the type of GSD. There are also many extrahepatic manifestations relating to hyperuricaemia, hyperlipidaemia and hypoglycaemic brain damage. If the hypoglycaemic episodes can be prevented progression of the liver disease is unlikely, except in GSD type IV, where cirrhosis is inevitable and leads to death within five years. Notably, this group of diseases is associated with multiple hepatic adenomas.

Gilbert's syndrome

Gilbert's syndrome, also known as hereditary non-haemolytic unconjugated hyperbilirubinaemia, is a condition resulting from a slight deficiency in the enzyme UDP glucuronyl transferase. This enzyme is responsible for the breakdown of bilirubin, and deficiency results in hyperbilirubinaemia. It is characterised by a mild, fluctuating increase in bilirubin, with rises often occurring during times of stress, fatigue or dehydration. It occurs in 1 in 20 people and is found more frequently in males. Diagnosis is often made just on liver function tests, when all tests except bilirubin are normal. This is a benign condition and has no implications for liver or biliary function.

Immune diseases of the liver

Autoimmune hepatitis (AIH)

Autoimmune hepatitis typically occurs in females, at puberty and between the ages of 40 and 70. It can also occur in males at any age. It may present in a number of ways: as a mild hepatitis, as a severe acute hepatitis or as established cirrhosis. The functioning capacity of the liver will vary depending on the stage of disease. The diagnosis of AIH is based on serum biochemistry, liver histology, and the presence of certain autoantibodies in the serum. Exclusion of other potential causes of hepatitis, e.g. hepatitis B or C, alcohol consumption, is needed before a definitive diagnosis can be made. There are no features that are specifically indicative of AIH, but it usually responds to treatment with corticosteroids. Once remission is induced azathioprine or mycophenolate are used to prevent relapse. If left untreated, AIH will gradually progress to cirrhosis and liver failure.

Primary biliary cirrhosis (PBC)

Primary biliary cirrhosis is an autoimmune chronic cholestatic disease of the liver. It is characterised by the progressive destruction of the small intrahepatic bile ducts and affects mainly middle-aged women. Patients are often asymptomatic on initial presentation and the diagnosis is based on abnormal liver function tests and the presence of antimitochondrial antibodies (M2 subtype). Initially cholestasis will develop that slowly progresses to cirrhosis and liver failure, when patients often have symptoms of uncontrollable pruritus, jaundice and severe lethargy. There is no cure, although ursodeoxycholic acid probably slows disease progression. Liver transplantation is often considered for these patients.

Primary sclerosing cholangitis (PSC)

Primary sclerosing cholangitis is characterised by inflammation, fibrosis and destruction of the intrahepatic and/or extrahepatic bile ducts. It results in a chronic cholestatic liver disease that may lead to liver cirrhosis. Cholangiocarcinoma occurs in approximately 10–30% of patients. PSC occurs more frequently in men between the ages of 20 and 40, with a male:female ratio of 2:1. It is often associated with inflammatory bowel disease, particularly chronic ulcerative colitis.

Sclerosing cholangitis in childhood is rare: it may overlap with autoimmune liver disease and may be secondary, for example, to Langerhans' cell histiocytosis.

Cancer

In adults the most common primary malignant tumour of the liver is hepatocellular carcinoma (HCC). In young children it is hepatoblastoma. HCC is strongly linked to cirrhosis, with 80% of patients having underlying cirrhosis. Patients with viral hepatitis or alcoholic liver disease have the greatest risk. Generally other primary malignant tumours in the liver are rare: they include cholangiocarcinoma, which is often associated with ulcerative colitis, angiosarcoma, fibrosarcoma and lymphoma. The liver is often the site of metastases of malignant tumours from elsewhere in the body, in particular the bowel.

Vascular abnormalities

Vascular abnormalities that may affect liver function can be split into disorders of the hepatic veins, of the hepatic arteries or of the portal vein system. The main disorders affecting the hepatic veins are the Budd–Chiari syndrome and veno-occlusive disease. Budd–Chiari syndrome develops when a blockage occurs in the large hepatic veins, as a result of either a sudden thrombotic event or a slow fibrous occlusion, often due to an underlying disorder of coagulation. This may occur suddenly, resulting in a presentation of subacute liver failure and ascites. Alternatively the occlusion may form slowly, with symptoms developing gradually over several months.

Veno-occlusive disease (VOD) differs from Budd–Chiari syndrome in that it consists of occlusive fibrosis of the small intrahepatic veins. VOD may present as either an acute form with sudden ascites, liver enlargement and rapidly rising bilirubin, or as a chronic form with fibrosis and cirrhosis. One of the main causes of VOD is the use of cyclophosphamide or alkalating agents during conditioning for bone marrow transplantation, where it occurs in up to 20% of cases. Other causes include irradiation, antineoplastic drugs, pyrrolizidine alkaloids and alcohol.

Biliary tract disorders

Disruption of bile flow may occur as a result of a number of disorders of the biliary tract, leading to the accumulation in the liver of bilirubin and hepatotoxic bile salts. This leads to inflammation of hepatocytes, scarring, and possibly cirrhosis. Obstruction of bile flow may be due to cholelithiasis (gallstones), cholangiocarcinoma (tumour in the biliary tree), cysts, or as a result of damage to the biliary tree in conditions such as primary biliary cirrhosis or cholangitis. It may also occur secondary to surgical or traumatic damage to the common bile duct. In children biliary atresia is one of the most common causes of chronic liver disease. It results from a congenital malformation of the extrahepatic bile ducts causing progressive jaundice, usually from the second week of life. If surgical intervention at this stage is not successful biliary atresia is likely to progress to fibrosis and cirrhosis. It is the most common indication for liver transplantation in children. Other congenital conditions affecting the biliary system include choledochal cysts. These occur as a result of a congenital abnormality of the common bile duct. Generally, by the age of two or three years (but sometimes much later) a cyst forms in the duct which may block bile flow. The patient presents with jaundice, and possibly abdominal pain and fever. If left untreated the accumulation of bile salts will damage the liver and may lead to cirrhosis and an increased risk of malignancy.

Other conditions associated with liver dysfunction

Diabetes mellitus

Liver disease is now recognised as a major complication of type 2 diabetes. Diabetes mellitus can lead to metabolic changes that alter normal hepatic and biliary function and structure. Type 2 diabetes is associated with an increased risk of a range of hepatobiliary diseases, including non-alcoholic fatty liver disease, cirrhosis, acute liver failure, hepatocellular carcinoma and cholelithiasis [22].

Pregnancy

It is normal to have a non-pathological increase in alkaline phosphatase during the third trimester of pregnancy owing to both a leakage of the enzyme from the placenta and an increase in maternal bone turnover. Albumin levels are generally reduced and serum transaminases and γ-glutamyl transpeptidase usually remain unchanged. Liver disease during pregnancy can be caused by conditions specific to pregnancy, such as intrahepatic cholestasis, acute fatty liver of pregnancy (AFLP), HELLP syndrome (haemolysis, elevated liver enzymes and low platelets) and cholelithiasis of pregnancy, or by liver diseases that are not related to pregnancy itself, such as viral hepatitis or cirrhosis. Elevation of liver enzymes is also commonly seen in pregnant women with pre-eclampsia and hyperemesis gravidarum.

Sickle cell disease

Patients with sickle cell disease often require blood transfusions. Most abnormalities of liver function in sickle cell patients result from infections transmitted by blood or as a result of iron overload from blood transfusion. Haemolysis due to sickle cell disease may result in increases in bilirubin. Patients may present with severe pain in the right upper quadrant and rapid enlargement of the liver as part of the hepatic sequestration syndrome.

Inflammatory bowel disease

Approximately 3–10% of patients with inflammatory bowel disease have some degree of liver abnormality. The spectrum of liver dysfunction associated with inflammatory bowel disease ranges from fatty changes to pericholangitis, sclerosing cholangitis, chronic active hepatitis and cirrhosis. Ulcerative colitis is more commonly associated with liver abnormality than Crohn's disease.

Congestive cardiac failure

Hepatomegaly is found in most patients with moderately severe heart failure. With progressive cardiac failure, jaundice occurs in about 25% of patients and may progress to necrosis, fibrosis and cirrhosis.

Sarcoidosis

Sarcoidosis is a systemic granulomatous disease of unknown aetiology. The liver is commonly involved, with evidence of granulomatous infiltration in up to 70% of cases. Symptoms are relatively uncommon and complications are unusual. Hepatomegaly and splenomegaly occur in

Table 3.6 Examples of some infections affecting the liver

Bacteria	Actinomycosis
	Brucellosis
	Chlamydia
	Escherichia coli
	Streptococcus sp.
Mycobacteria	Tuberculosis
	Leprosy
Protozoa	Malaria
	Toxoplasmosis
	Giardiasis
Fungi	Aspergillosis
	Candida
	Cryptococcus
Trematodes	Schistosomiasis

approximately 25% of patients. Elevations in alkaline phosphatase occur commonly, although jaundice is rare. Liver function usually remains unaffected.

Infections

Organisms other than the viruses discussed earlier can cause acute liver infections, such as *Leptospira icterohaemorrhagia*, which causes Weil's disease, fungal infections caused by *Candida* species or aspergillosis, and schistosomiasis caused by trematodes. A number of systemic infections may also affect the liver, leading to jaundice, abnormal liver function tests or even acute liver failure. Table 3.6 lists some of the infective organisms that have been associated with liver disease.

Key points

- A wide range of conditions may cause liver disease.
- Liver disease does not necessarily mean liver dysfunction.
- Liver disease may be classified as cholestatic, hepatocellular or cirrhotic.
- Liver disease may be acute, with the history of onset of less than six months, or chronic, occurring over periods greater than six months.
- Viral infections and drug reactions are leading causes of acute liver disease in both adults and children.
- Alcohol consumption is the leading cause of chronic liver disease in adults. Biliary atresia is a leading cause of chronic liver disease in children.

Guided further reading

Benjaminov FS, Heathcote J. Liver disease in pregnancy. *Am J Gastroenterol* 2004; 99: 2479–2488.

Kelly DA (ed) (2004) *Diseases of the Liver and Biliary System in Children,* 2nd edn. Oxford: Blackwell.

Kennedy PTF, O'Grady J. Diseases of the liver. Chronic liver disease. *Hosp Pharmacist* 2002; 9: 137–144.

Richardson P, O'Grady J. Diseases of the liver. Acute liver disease. *Hosp Pharmacist* 2002; 9: 131–136.

Section 14: Gastroenterology. In: Weatherall DJ, Ledingham JG, Warrell DA (eds) *Oxford Textbook of Medicine,* 3rd edn. Oxford: Oxford Medical Publications, 1996, 2014–2136.

References

1. Richardson P, O'Grady J. Diseases of the liver. Acute liver disease. *Hosp Pharmacist* 2002; 9: 1336.
2. Grant BF, Dufour MC, Harford TC. Epidemiology of alcoholic liver disease. *Semin Liver Dis* 1988; 8: 15.
3. WHO. Regional Office for Europe. [online] 2003 [accessed 30.10.2005] Available from: http://data.euro.who.int/cisid/
4. Becker U, Deis A, Sorensen TI, *et al.* Prediction of risk of liver disease by alcohol intake, sex, and age: a prospective population study. *Hepatology* 1996; 23: 1029.
5. Tuys A, Pequignot G. Great risk of ascitic cirrhosis in females in relation to alcohol consumption. *Int J Epidemiol* 1984; 13: 53–57.
6. Grove J, Daly AK, Bassendine MF, *et al.* Association of tumour necrosis factor promoter polymorphism with susceptibility to alcoholic steatohepatitis. *Hepatology* 1997; 26: 143–146.
7. Jarvelainen HA, Orpana A, Perola M, *et al.* Promoter polymorphism of the CD14 endotoxin receptor gene as a risk factor for alcoholic liver disease. *Hepatology* 2001; 33: 1148–1153.
8. Bosron WF, Ehrig T, Li TK. Genetic factors in alcohol metabolism and alcoholism. *Semin Liver Dis* 1993; 13: 126–135.
9. Pares A, Barrera JM, Caballeria J, *et al.* Hepatitis C virus antibodies in chronic alcoholic patients: association with severity of liver injury. *Hepatology* 1990; 12: 1295–1299.
10. McSween RNM, Burt AD. Histologic spectrum of alcoholic liver disease. *Semin Liver Dis* 1986; 3: 221–232.
11. Galambos JT. Natural history of alcoholic hepatitis. 3. Histological changes. *Gastroenterology* 1972; 63: 1026–1035.
12. Lee WM. Hepatitis B virus infection. *N Engl J Med* 1997; 336: 1733–1745.
13. Buendia MA. Hepatitis B viruses and carcinogenesis. *Biomed Pharmacother* 1998; 52: 34–43.
14. Liaw YF, Chen YC, Sheen I, *et al.* Impact of acute hepatitis C virus superinfection in patients with chronic hepatitis B virus infection. *Gastroenterology* 2004; 126: 1024–1029.
15. World Health Organization. Fact Sheet 164. Revised 2000. Available from www.who.int/mediacentre/factsheets/fs164/en/index.html
16. Benjaminov FS, Heathcote J. Liver disease in pregnancy. *Am J Gastroenterol* 2004; 99: 2479–2488.
17. Brunt EM. Nonalcoholic steatohepatitis. *Semin Liver Dis* 2004; 24: 3–20.
18. Marchesini G, Bugianesi E, Forlani G, *et al.* Nonalcoholic fatty liver, steatohepatitis, and the metabolic syndrome. *Hepatology* 2003; 37: 917–923.
19. Wanless IR, Lentz JS. Fatty liver hepatitis (steatohepatitis) and obesity: an autopsy study with analysis of risk factors. *Hepatology* 1990; 12: 1106–1110.
20. Zimmerman HJ. Hepatotoxicity. The adverse effects of drugs and other chemicals in the liver, 2nd edn. Philadelphia: Lippincott Williams & Wilkins, 1999.
21. Mason P. Cystic fibrosis – the disease. *Hosptal Pharmacist* 2005; 12: 201–207.
22. Tolman KG, Fonseca V, Tan MH, *et al.* Narrative review: hepatobiliary disease in type 2 diabetes mellitus. *Ann Intern Med* 2004; 141: 946–956.

4

Assessing liver function

Catherine Hughes

Objectives

By the end of this chapter the reader should be able to:

- Explain why there is no simple method of calculating a patient's liver function.
- Be able to make an assessment of a patient's liver function status by interpreting:
  - Liver function tests (LFTs)
  - Other test results
  - Diagnosis
  - Signs and symptoms.
- Be able to determine whether a patient's liver function needs to be taken into account in the choice of drug and dosage.

Introduction

Impaired liver function may affect the handling of some drugs because of changes in pharmacokinetics or pharmacodynamics. For example, reduced drug elimination by the liver may cause higher serum levels, which in turn lead to increased therapeutic effect and the potential for increased side effects. Depending on the clinical circumstances, a patient's liver function may need to be estimated to assist in making appropriate initial drug choices or changes to existing therapy.

Unlike in renal medicine, there is no simple method of estimating liver function because:

- There is no single marker, such as the glomerular filtration rate (GFR) in renal medicine.
- Every drug is handled differently in patients with different liver conditions.
- Often little is known about the pharmacokinetics and pharmacodynamics of an individual drug in impaired liver function.

This chapter will look at how a judgement can be made about the extent of a patient's liver dysfunction. These tools can be used along with other chapters in the book to assist in making the correct choice of drug and dosage for each patient.

It has already been stated that no one marker can be used to estimate liver function. A combination of factors need to be considered to give an accurate estimate of an individual's liver function (Figure 4.1). These are:

- Liver function tests (LFTs) and other test results.
- Diagnosis (including the presence or absence of fibrosis, cirrhosis and hepatic decompensation).
- The patient's signs and symptoms of liver disease.

Any of the above used in isolation may lead to an inaccurate assessment and hence potentially inappropriate drug use. A patient with the same LFTs as another may have very different signs and symptoms,

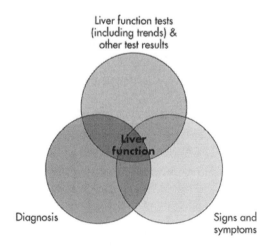

Figure 4.1 Factors to be considered when estimating liver function.

which may lead to a different judgement about the liver function and hence the choice of drug or dose. For example, an obese man with a long-standing alanine transferase (ALT) of 100 IU/L (reference range up to 35 IU/L) and no other abnormal results or signs of liver disease may have a diagnosis of fatty liver disease. This suggests there will be no effect on liver function and hence the ALT of 100 IU/L in this case would not be of concern and not affect drug choice. Conversely, a second patient with an ALT of 100 IU/L which has been increasing over a period of three weeks, albeit with no other abnormal results, has spider naevi (vascular changes on the skin; see later in the chapter for further details), which indicates a chronic liver condition and may suggest that this patient has cirrhosis and the increase in ALT is because the liver is decompensating. For this patient there will almost certainly be altered drug handling, which will affect drug choice and dose.

It is clear from these examples that it is essential to be able to assess accurately which patients need to have their liver function taken into consideration when prescribing.

The following sections of this chapter look at the individual components of LFTs and how they need to be considered as a group, over time, to interpret them effectively. Also discussed is what other test results, signs and symptoms indicate, along with methodologies, such as Child–Pugh, which are used to compare individuals' liver function.

The ultimate aim of the chapter is to provide a guide to determine which patients should be of concern regarding drug choice and dose, and those which are not.

Liver function tests (LFTs)

Introduction

The LFT is a blood test to determine serum levels of a group of constituents, usually:

- Transaminases: alanine transferase (ALT) and/or aspartate transferase (AST)
- Alkaline phosphatase (alk phos, ALP)
- Bilirubin
- Albumin
- Total protein (in some laboratories).

Serum γ-glutamyl transpeptidase (GGT) is also occasionally included as part of the standard test by some laboratories. Although the clotting screen does not form part of the LFT, it is essential to consider it when assessing a patient's liver function. For the purposes of this chapter, when LFT is referred to it will include the clotting screen.

LFTs have a limited role in assessing the degree of liver function when used in isolation. Contrary to what the name suggests, the LFT alone does not inform us of the function of the liver *per se*. One reason for this is that none of the constituents of the test are specific for the liver, and therefore a change in a level does not necessarily indicate a change in the liver. A patient with liver damage may have normal LFTs because the disease is not severe enough to affect the result, or the liver is still functioning well despite being diseased.

There are some key points to consider when interpreting a patient's LFTs:

- Generally, a result which is twice the upper limit of normal (ULN) is considered to be abnormal. However, bear in mind that some or all the values may be within a normal range even if a patient has liver dysfunction.
- If a patient has liver dysfunction, it is usual that more than one of the LFTs will be abnormal.
- All of the constituents of the LFT can be altered by changes not related to the liver.
- Do not look at one LFT result in isolation: it is important to look at trends over hours, days, weeks or months (depending on whether the picture is acute or chronic).
- Check the reference ranges used by the laboratory that carried out the test, as these can vary.

Background information on individual LFTs

Transaminases

- Alanine transferase (ALT) (formerly known as serum glutamic oxaloacetic transaminase: SGOT)
- Aspartate transferase (AST) (formerly known as serum glutamic pyruvic transaminases: SGPT)
- Usual reference range for adults and children: 0–40 IU/L.

ALT and AST are enzymes released from hepatocytes when they are damaged, resulting in high serum levels when there is hepatocellular injury.

AST is also found in large concentrations in the heart, pancreas, kidney, lung, muscle and red blood cells. ALT is found in other tissues, but is present in much larger quantities in the liver, making it more specific to the liver than AST. Other conditions, such as acute cardiac failure, may cause ALT and AST levels to rise significantly as a result of cardiac muscle damage and liver cell hypoxia. AST and ALT levels tend to rise and fall at the same time.

In an acute hepatocellular injury, such as following a paracetamol overdose, there may be significant damage over a short period. This results in a marked increase in the AST and ALT levels (which can be in the thousands) due to massive hepatocyte damage or death. The converse can occur with chronic severe disease, where the hepatocyte mass has reduced to such an extent that the AST and ALT levels have returned to normal owing to the reduction in hepatocyte numbers able to release the enzyme (i.e. a false normal result). In fatty liver, ALT and AST levels are likely to be up to three times ULN, whereas in hepatitis ALT and AST levels can range from nearly normal to in the hundreds, depending on how acute the condition is.

Bilirubin

- Usual reference range for adults and children: 5–21 µmol/L.

Bilirubin is produced by the transformation of haem (mainly from the destruction of red blood cells) via biliverdin (see Figure 2.8). This takes place in the liver, spleen and bone marrow. Bilirubin is transported to the liver in the serum attached to albumin, and at this stage is unconjugated. It is insoluble in water and hence cannot be excreted in this form. Hepatocytes transform unconjugated bilirubin into a water-soluble conjugated form which is excreted via the bile into the intestine. Here, some is converted to urobilinogen and excreted by the kidneys, the majority being converted to stercobilin and excreted in the faeces.

Total bilirubin (both conjugated and unconjugated fractions) is measured as part of the standard LFT. The conjugated and unconjugated bilirubin can be measured as separate fractions, which can be useful as part of a diagnosis for some conditions, e.g. obstructive jaundice (high conjugated fraction) or haemolytic anaemia and congenital hyperbilirubinaemias such as Gilbert's syndrome (high unconjugated fraction). In haemolytic anaemias, such as sickle cell disease, the rate of red blood cell destruction is greater than the liver's capacity to conjugate the bilirubin, and so the body is unable to excrete it.

A serum total bilirubin level in excess of 50 µmol/L can produce clinical jaundice in adults. In neonates a level of 80 µmol/L or above can show jaundice. Bilirubin may be raised in cholestasis, often alongside the biliary tract enzymes, alkaline phosphatase and GGT. It can also be raised in acute liver failure, potentially in the hundreds, owing to the liver's inability to conjugate the bilirubin, preventing its excretion. In chronic compensated cirrhotic patients with no cholestasis, the bilirubin may be normal. For further information on bilirubin, see Chapter 2.

Alkaline phosphatase

- Reference ranges: Depending on the assay method used, the reference range for alkaline phosphatase varies. Always ensure you are using the right reference range for the laboratory when interpreting results. See Table 4.1 for examples.

The term alkaline phosphatase describes a group of isoenzymes which are released from different parts of the body. The hepatic alkaline phosphatase is produced by hepatocytes. Production is increased when there is damage to the biliary tract, hence a raised alkaline phosphatase level can be a marker for biliary damage, obstruction or cholestasis. This can be intra- or extrahepatic in origin, and causes include drugs, tumours and gallstones. Drugs and gallstones can cause alkaline phosphatase to rise up to ten times ULN, and tumours can cause it to rise to three times ULN.

However, other isoenzymes of alkaline phosphatase are found in parts of the body such as bone, kidney, intestine and placenta, hence an isolated raised alkaline phosphatase may not be associated with liver dysfunction. In late pregnancy, alkaline phosphatase can increase to three times ULN, which may persist for several months after delivery, particularly if the mother is breastfeeding, owing to bone effects. In

Table 4.1 Examples of usual reference ranges for alkaline phosphatase

	Alkaline phosphatase reference range (IU/L)	
Age range	*Assay method one*	*Assay method two*
Adults	0–300	0–120
Adolescent	200–600	0–450
Child 1–9 years old	200–500	0–350
Child 1 month to 1 year	100–400	0–450
Neonate	120–500	0–450

Reference ranges may vary depending on gender and age group.

Paget's disease the level can range from normal to up to ten times the ULN, depending on the location and severity of the disease. Increased bone turnover in adolescents means the normal range of alkaline phosphatase is twice that of adults. In these cases there is no liver involvement. Some laboratories can measure the individual isoenzymes to give a more accurate assessment of the origin of the enzyme release; however, this is seldom necessary, as the diagnosis can be made by looking at other factors, e.g. a raised GGT can confirm that a raised alkaline phosphatase is of hepatobiliary origin.

γ-Glutamyl transpeptidase (GGT, gamma-GT, γ-GT)

- Usual reference range for adults and children: 0–50 IU/L.

GGT does not usually form part of the standard LFTs in most laboratories. It is an enzyme found in hepatocytes and biliary epithelial cells, and also in kidney, pancreas, intestine and prostate. It has a higher sensitivity for indicating a problem of liver origin than alkaline phosphatase, but tends to follow a similar pattern. It is released in all types of liver dysfunction and therefore cannot generally be used to differentiate between types. However, a raised GGT with an isolated raised alkaline phosphatase can be suggestive of cholestasis. GGT levels can be ten to 20 times normal in cholestatic disease.

An isolated raised GGT can also occur in alcohol abuse. In alcoholics, levels can vary significantly from normal to in excess of 20 times ULN. If raised, it may return to normal within two to five weeks of stopping drinking, but the maintenance of a high level does not necessarily indicate a continuation of abuse, as there may be other factors that influence the level, such as the presence of liver disease.

GGT levels may also be raised in patients taking enzyme-inducing drugs such as phenytoin or rifampicin, where levels can be commonly measured at twice ULN and potentially up to five times. Those with concomitant diseases, such as diabetes mellitus, can have GGT levels up to three times ULN, which may be due to a fatty liver.

Plasma proteins

The liver is responsible for manufacturing many plasma proteins, including albumin, α_1-antitrypsin, α-feto protein and prothrombin. The measurement of total plasma protein is of little value in determining liver function, as values may be normal despite disturbances in the production of individual proteins. The two proteins which are of significance when determining liver function – albumin and pro-thrombin – are discussed below.

Albumin

• Usual reference range for adults and children: 34–45 g/L.

The majority of albumin in the blood has been manufactured by the liver; accordingly, serum albumin is a marker of the liver's synthetic capacity. Albumin has a half-life of about 20 days and therefore is used as an indicator of chronic disease. In cirrhosis, albumin production can fall by more than 50%, leading to serum levels as low as 20 g/L. A patient with acute liver failure is likely to have a normal albumin level initially.

When interpreting a patient's albumin level, possible extrahepatic causes for low levels should be considered, for example a reduction in albumin production associated with malnutrition and malignancy, or increased albumin loss seen in inflammatory bowel disease and nephrotic syndrome.

Prothrombin

Prothrombin, also produced by the liver, is a clotting factor essential for normal coagulation. Prothrombin is one of the vitamin K-dependent clotting factors, which means that it has no coagulating properties unless vitamin K is present to transform it. Consequently, reduced intake or absorption of fat-soluble vitamin K will increase the time taken for blood to clot.

Clotting screen

The clotting screen, which includes prothrombin time (PT) and inter-national normalised ratio (INR), is not part of the standard LFT but is essential for the assessment of a patient's liver function. As the liver is responsible for synthesising clotting factors this is the key marker for determining and monitoring liver function trends.

Prothrombin time (PT)

• Usual reference range for adults and children: 12–16 seconds.

PT is a laboratory test which measures the time taken for a clot to form. If there is a reduction in prothrombin, one of the other clotting factors or the availability of vitamin K, the time it takes to clot will be prolonged, i.e. PT will be increased. If the prolongation is secondary to vitamin K deficiency then the administration of 10–20 mg of intravenous vitamin K will correct the clotting time within 12–24 hours. If the PT is not corrected by the administration of vitamin K it is likely that the coagulopathy is due to reduced liver synthesis of clotting factors, a congenital deficiency of one or more clotting factors, or another cause such as anticoagulant therapy or severe malnutrition.

In chronic liver disease, PT may increase over a period of weeks or months to values up to about 30 seconds as the liver decompensates. In patients with acute liver failure the values may increase to over 100 seconds within a few hours.

PT is increasingly being replaced by INR, as it is a more accurate method of comparing clotting across laboratories.

International normalised ratio (INR)

Usual reference range for adults and children: 0.9–1.2.

The INR is the PT value expressed as a ratio when compared to a control value. An INR above 1.2 is regarded as abnormal. In chronic liver disease the INR may increase over a period of weeks or months to values up to about 2.5 as the liver decompensates. In patients with acute liver failure the values may increase to over 10 within a few hours. See Table 4.2 for a summary of LFT background information.

Interpreting LFTs and their trends

So far this chapter has looked at each of the constituents of LFTs; however, to be able to interpret LFTs accurately, all of the components should be considered together as this may affect the overall assessment. To take that one step further, it is not just one LFT result that should be studied, but a series of LFTs over a period of hours, days, weeks or months (depending on the rate of change), to indicate whether the liver function is stable, improving or deteriorating.

Table 4.3 summarises the potential extent of change in each individual LFT for an example patient with compensated chronic liver disease, decompensated chronic liver disease, hepatitis, hyperacute liver failure and cholestasis. This is a snapshot of the changes that may occur in these conditions; however, if each patient's results were observed over time a range of results would be seen.

Below is a description of how LFT trends may change over time for each of the patient groups.

Table 4.2 Summary of liver function test background information

Test	Where found/produced	Normal range (vary between hospitals)	Possible implications when level abnormal
Transaminases: Alanine aminotransferase (ALT)	Liver, heart, skeletal muscle	0–40 IU/L	Raised levels indicate hepatocyte damage/necrosis ALT is more liver specific but has a longer half-life, so less sensitive
Aspartate aminotransferase (AST)		0–40 IU/L	May be normal in compensated liver cirrhosis
Alkaline phosphatase (ALP)	Liver, kidney, bone, placenta, intestine, biliary epithelia	30–300 IU/L (higher in children due to increased bone growth)	Raised levels may indicate biliary inflammation/obstruction, malignant infiltration, cirrhosis, bone destruction, Paget's disease
Gamma-glutamyl transpeptidase (GGT, γ-GT)	Biliary epithelia, hepatocytes	0–50 IU/L	Raised in many forms of liver disease and in enzyme induction, e.g. alcohol or certain medicines
Bilirubin	Produced from haemoglobin during degradation of erythrocytes. Found in bile	5–21 µmol/L	Raised in hepatocyte dysfunction, biliary obstruction and haemolysis
Albumin	Synthesised in the liver	34–45 g/L	Low levels indicate chronic liver disease (poor synthetic function), malnutrition or increased loss, e.g. nephropathy
Clotting: Prothrombin time (PT)/international normalised ratio (INR)	Coagulation factors synthesised in the liver	PT <16 seconds INR <1.2	Prolonged (significant elevation PT >3 seconds above normal range or INR >1.2) in chronic and acute liver disease Useful prognostic indicator of impending/recovering liver failure (acute/decompensated liver disease)

Table 4.3 Examples of usual patterns of LFTs for patients with different liver conditions

Type of dysfunction / LFT	ALT/AST	Alk Phos	Bilirubin	Albumin	INR/PT
Compensated chronic liver disease	↔ to ↑↑	↔ to ↑	↔ to ↑↑↑↑	↔ to ↓	↔ to INR 1.4
Decompensated chronic liver disease	↔ to ↑↑	↔ to ↑↑	↔ to ↑↑↑↑	↓ to ↓↓	↑
Hepatitis	↑ to ↑↑↑↑	↔ to ↑↑	↑ to ↑↑↑	↔ to ↓	↔ to ↑
Hyperacute liver failure	↑↑↑↑	↔ to ↑↑	↔ to ↑↑↑	↔	↑↑↑
Cholestasis	↔	↑↑ or ↑↑↑	↑↑ or ↑↑↑	↔	↔

↔	Within reference range.
↑	Up to twice upper limit of normal (ULN).
↑↑	Up to three times ULN.
↑↑↑	Up to ten times ULN.
↑↑↑↑	Up to 20 times ULN.
↑↑↑↑↑	More than 20 times ULN.
↓	75% of normal.
↓↓	50% of normal.

NB These examples are at one point in time, it is important to consider the trends of the LFTs as discussed in the chapter.

This is a guide to how LFTs may change with different liver conditions. It is important that reference ranges for the laboratory and age of the patient are used.

Compensated chronic liver disease

If the patient has severe end-stage disease and only limited numbers of functioning hepatocytes the ALT may be normal. In the initial stages of the disease while hepatocyte damage was at a peak, the ALT will have risen to up to three times ULN. Gradually, over months or years, however, it will have reduced to a normal level, but this does not indicate an improvement in the condition. The residual liver function can be estimated by looking at the albumin and clotting screen. For a patient with compensated liver function, the albumin level will be normal or slightly reduced and the clotting normal or slightly increased.

Depending on the nature of the chronic liver disease, the biliary tract may or may not be affected, and hence bilirubin and alkaline phosphatase may be normal or raised. For example, a patient with primary biliary cirrhosis (PBC) can have an alkaline phosphatase and bilirubin raised to twice ULN. Where there is biliary involvement there is the potential for reduced fat-soluble vitamin absorption. Hence a raised alkaline phosphatase may have occurred over time owing to decreased vitamin D absorption affecting bone development, rather than being associated with the liver. Likewise, the clotting may be abnormal because of vitamin K deficiency.

Decompensated chronic liver disease

The results may be similar to those of the patient with compensated chronic liver disease described above, with the exception of albumin and clotting screen. The synthetic function of the liver will have deteriorated as it can no longer compensate, and therefore the albumin will be reduced and PT and INR raised. The INR is a particularly sensitive method of detecting impending decompensation of liver function in a previously stable patient. It is also used to determine whether liver function is improving. The increase in INR can occur over a period of days or weeks, with albumin decreasing over a few weeks owing to its longer half-life.

Hepatitis

The causes of hepatitis are varied, as are their effects on liver function. Viruses, such as hepatitis B (HBV), follow different patterns in individuals. For example, following exposure to HBV, 2–10% of adults and nearly 100% of newborns will develop chronic hepatitis, which can lead to cirrhosis and hepatocellular carcinoma. Those who do not develop chronic hepatitis will have cleared the virus from the body entirely, leaving no residual long-term damage. Autoimmune hepatitis may go through periods of active and inactive disease over months or years, and hence LFTs will change as the condition waxes and wanes. Drug-induced hepatitis can be an acute condition which, if the patient recovers, leaves no residual effects as the damaged hepatocytes regenerate.

Hepatitis is inflammation of the liver and therefore the ALT and AST will increase to some extent as they are released from the damaged hepatocytes. Hepatitis can be an acute condition where the damage and transaminase increase occur over 28 days or less, and levels can be measured in the hundreds. A more chronic condition would show a rise over months or years, with lower levels than the acute condition. The magnitude of the rise in ALT and AST depends on the extent of cell damage, which will also determine whether other LFTs change. It may be that the liver's functional capacity is unaffected and hence no other LFTs change, or that the cell death is severe enough to affect the synthetic function and hence INR rises and albumin reduces. Additionally, it may be that the conjugating capacity of the liver is reduced, and hence bilirubin can rise to several hundred. If this does occur it tends to lag behind the rise in transaminases and may continue to increase even after they have started to recover. It can take several weeks before the bilirubin returns to normal.

Hyperacute liver failure

Hyperacute liver failure is where encephalopathy occurs within seven days of the onset of jaundice and coagulopathy is present. This can occur as a result of a drug-induced reaction, such as a paracetamol overdose, metabolic conditions including Wilson's disease and neonatal haemochromatosis, or viruses such as HBV. In all cases, the ALT and AST would rise rapidly over the initial 24–48 hours and can be in excess of 10 000 IU/L. If the liver starts to recover, it can reach a peak at around seven days and then gradually reduce to normal over the next two to three weeks. The clotting screen is the best indicator of damage and prognosis. The INR will increase dramatically during the initial 24–48 hours, potentially to levels of ten or more. The level is measured every six hours at this stage and indicates recovery of the liver as it begins to fall. The INR should return to normal in about two weeks. Bilirubin can be in the hundreds and lags behind the increase in ALT, AST and INR as it gradually rises over the initial few days, reaching a peak around day seven. Should the liver begin to recover, bilirubin will decline over the following few weeks, with jaundice remaining for up to six weeks.

If the liver continues to deteriorate, death is likely within a few days unless an emergency transplant can be performed.

Cholestasis

Cholestasis refers to the reduced excretion of bile salts – not necessarily bilirubin – from the liver. In cholestatic patients the liver is generally functioning normally and hence ALT, AST and albumin are normal unless the condition has progressed towards cirrhosis. The INR may be raised as an indicator of vitamin K deficiency caused by malabsorption. In cholestasis it is the biliary tract that is affected, and therefore the biliary tract enzymes, alkaline phosphatase and GGT, and bilirubin may be increased as their removal through the biliary tract is reduced. Gallstones can cause bilirubin levels to rise to up to 20 times ULN, as well as an elevation in alkaline phosphatase, which occurs over a period of days or weeks and reduces over a few days when the blockage is removed. A more insidious condition such as primary biliary cirrhosis (PBC) causes bilirubin and alkaline phosphatase to rise over many months or years and to go through periods of increasing and decreasing as the condition waxes and wanes. Some intrahepatic cholestases have normal bilirubin because the mechanism for excreting bilirubin from hepatocytes into biliary canaliculi may be unaffected, whereas that used to excrete bile salts is impaired.

Other tests carried out in suspected hepatobiliary dysfunction

Ultrasound

An ultrasound is the first radiological investigation to be carried out when hepatobiliary dysfunction is suspected.

Liver ultrasound

Ultrasound can be used to estimate the size of the liver. A small atrophied nodular liver suggests cirrhosis, and a large hypertrophied liver is inflamed or fatty. Liver lesions can be visualised, which may be malignant and large enough to affect the function of the remaining cells.

Ultrasound of the gallbladder

The size and contents of the gallbladder can be visualised on ultrasound. This can be used to assess cholecystitis and gallstones, but tells us little about liver function *per se*.

A fasting ultrasound should show a full gallbladder, which would be emptied when the patient next ate a meal. If the fasted gallbladder is small and irregular bile may not be flowing into it from the liver, which may suggest obstruction or, in infants, biliary atresia.

Ultrasound of the bile ducts

Dilatation of both the intrahepatic and extrahepatic ducts and the common bile duct is clearly seen by ultrasound, indicating obstruction, e.g. by gallstones or tumour.

Doppler

Doppler examination can be carried out during an ultrasound investigation. Doppler is used to measure the direction and speed of blood flow in vessels and the presence of any collateral vessels. In portal hypertension, the collateral vessels can have either flow in both directions or a total reversal of flow.

Liver biopsy

A biopsy is often required to make a diagnosis of most types of liver disease. A specimen of liver can be used to identify fibrosis, cirrhosis, cholestasis and hepatitis, both acute and chronic, and tumours. Biochemical measurements can also be taken from a biopsy specimen to determine iron and copper content, virology, microbiology and haematology (e.g. increased numbers of eosinophils in a drug-induced cause). The biopsy can give an indication of the extent of the liver damage. See Chapter 3 for slides of liver biopsies.

Computed tomography (CT)

CT is a technique that uses ionising radiation and computer processing to generate cross-sectional three-dimensional images of the internal organs. In assessment of the hepatobiliary tract both an oral contrast agent and an intravenous contrast medium are required to visualise the bowel and blood vessels, respectively. In the context of hepatobiliary disease, CT is particularly useful in assessing the extent of mass lesions.

Endoscopic retrograde cholangiopancreatography (ERCP)

Contrast medium is injected into the bile ducts via an endoscopic tube. X-rays are then used to visualise the pancreas and biliary tree. Gallstones can be removed during ERCP and stents can be inserted to widen narrowed bile ducts, which may be the cause of jaundice.

Magnetic resonance imaging (MRI)

An MRI scan is a radiological technique that uses magnetism, radio waves and a computer to produce images of body structures. MRI can provide sectional views of the body in multiple planes and does not involve ionising radiation. This technique is used to provide detail about liver tumours and portal vessels.

Magnetic resonance cholangiopancreatography (MRCP)

MRCP visualises the biliary and pancreatic system and is used to identify obstruction. It uses MRI and the inherent contrast properties of bile and pancreatic fluids to produce the image, and therefore does not require the injection of contrast media. It is used as an alternative to ERCP as it is non-invasive and can be used for patients with a history of allergy to iodine.

Hepatic angiography and venography

The hepatic vessels may be visualised by conventional angiography or venography. These are invasive techniques requiring the injection of contrast media into the artery or vein via catheters during radiographic screening. Stenoses or occlusions are identified, e.g. occlusion of the hepatic veins in Budd–Chiari syndrome.

Percutaneous transhepatic cholangiography (PTC)

PTC is a technique where contrast medium is injected into the common bile duct via a needle inserted through the skin in the right upper quadrant. X-ray images are used to identify strictures or obstructions in the biliary tree.

Hepatobiliary scintigraphy (HIDA)

A HIDA scan assesses the patency and function of the biliary tree. A radiolabelled isotope, technetium-99m (^{99m}Tc), is injected intravenously and actively taken up by hepatocytes and excreted into biliary canali-culi. Uptake and excretion into bile is visualised by placing a Geiger counter-type device on the patient's abdomen. HIDA is used to diagnose problems with the gallbladder and biliary tree, often where ultrasound has been inconclusive, e.g. suspected bile leaks after trauma or surgery, or the investigation of biliary atresia in infants.

If the ^{99m}Tc is absorbed by the liver but not secreted into the bile ducts, there is probably a complete obstruction of the ducts exiting the liver. When the ^{99m}Tc fails to appear in the gallbladder but is detected in the intestine, there is probably an obstruction of the cystic duct lead-ing to and from the gallbladder. Finally, if the ^{99m}Tc appears outside the liver, bile ducts, gallbladder or intestine, there is probably a bile leak from the bile ducts or gallbladder.

Diagnosis

The diagnosis is a key factor in interpreting patients' LFTs and assess-ing the degree of liver dysfunction. A patient may have a diagnosis of cirrhosis secondary to autoimmune hepatitis, with normal LFTs and no signs and symptoms of liver disease. Even though their LFTs are normal the diagnosis indicates that they have severe liver disease. In this case it is well compensated; however, there is a possibility that their liver func-tion could be compromised, which may require an alternative choice of drug. For example, a particularly hepatotoxic drug, such as methotrex-ate, should be avoided where possible. See Chapter 3 for more details on the causes of liver disease.

Signs and symptoms of liver dysfunction

Presenting signs and symptoms are among the three key factors in assessing the extent of the patient's liver function. Some assist in the diagnosis and indicate prognosis, whereas others are non-specific in terms of diagnosis but have a big impact on the patient's quality of life (Table 4.4).

Signs and symptoms suggestive of impaired liver function

Jaundice

In adults, yellowing of the skin or jaundice usually occur when serum bilirubin is higher than 50 µmol/L. In neonates, a bilirubin level in

Table 4.4 Signs and symptoms of liver dysfunction

Signs and symptoms suggestive of liver dysfunction	Less specific signs and symptoms of liver dysfunction
Jaundice	Malnutrition
Pale stool and dark urine	Peripheral oedema
Gynaecomastia	Bruising and bleeding
Spider naevi	Testicular atrophy
Ascites	White nails
Oesophageal and gastric varices	Splenomegaly
Hepatic encephalopathy	Palmar erythema
Dupuytren's contracture	Fatigue/malaise
Finger clubbing	Abdominal and right upper quadrant pain
Pruritus	Muscle cramps

It should be noted that, in isolation, few signs or symptoms are specific for liver dysfunction.

excess of 80 µmol/L is required before jaundice appears. Jaundice may be caused by high serum levels of conjugated or unconjugated bilirubin. It can occur with acute or chronic liver diseases, such as acute hepatitis or cirrhosis. The presence of jaundice does not give an indication of liver function. Benign liver conditions, such as Gilbert's syndrome, can cause jaundice as a result of high unconjugated bilirubin, but liver function is unaffected. Also, non-liver-related conditions such as haemolysis can cause jaundice.

Pale stools and dark urine

Pale stools are a sign of biliary obstruction. Normally, bile is secreted into the intestine, where the majority is converted to the faecal pigment stercobilin. If there is a biliary obstruction bile secretion is reduced and this conversion cannot take place, and so the stools do not have the usual coloration. Where there is complete obstruction, such as in biliary atresia, the stools may be white.

Dark urine occurs in obstructive jaundice because the water-soluble conjugated bilirubin cannot be excreted through the faeces. Excretion from the body is compensated for by increased kidney elimination, and hence the urine is a darker colour than normal.

Steatorrhoea

Steatorrhoea is excess fat in the stool, otherwise known as fatty stools. In cholestasis and bile salt disease this is due to a bile salt deficiency in the digestive tract, which causes a reduction in fat absorption from the gut. It can also occur with drugs such as orlistat. Steatorrhoea is associated with a reduction in the absorption of fat-soluble vitamins, and there is often a need to supplement.

Gynaecomastia

This is an enlargement of male breast tissue. It occurs in chronic liver disease as a result of reduced oestrogen degradation by the liver. It is a relatively specific sign of severe chronic liver disease and suggests impaired metabolic function and hence potentially an impaired ability to metabolise some drugs. However, some of these patients may also be taking spironolactone for ascites, which can cause gynaecomastia as an adverse effect as it inhibits testosterone production. Consequently, it may be difficult to determine whether it is an adverse effect of spirono-lactone or liver impairment that is implicated.

Spider naevi

These are associated with vascular changes that occur as a result of long-term liver disease. Although not specific for liver disease, they are commonly found on the torso of patients with chronic liver disease and may indicate impaired liver function (Figure 4.2).

Ascites

This is the presence of excess fluid in the peritoneal cavity, leading to a swollen abdomen (Figure 4.3). The accumulation of ascitic fluid represents a state of sodium excess in the body. Patients often present with hyponatraemia, but this is thought to be due to the dilutional effect of excess water rather than to low sodium. There are three theories of the cause of ascites formation. The underfill theory suggests that there is a reduction in circulating plasma volume as a result of accu-mulation in the splanchnic area due to vascular dilatation in portal hypertension. This activates the plasma renin, aldosterone and sym-pathetic nervous systems, which leads to sodium and water retention by the kidneys.

The overfill theory suggests that renal sodium retention occurs in the presence of increased plasma volume.

The peripheral arterial vasodilatation theory includes compon-ents of both of the other theories. It suggests that initially portal -

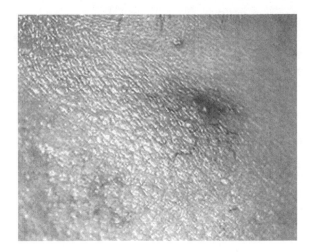

Figure 4.2 Spider naevi. Reproduced with permission from Fitzpatrick TB (1997), *Color Atlas and Synopsis of Clinical Dermatology*, 3rd edn. McGraw Hill.

hypertension leads to vasodilatation, which causes decreased effective arterial blood volume and causes the activation of the renin–angiotensin system. This leads to renal vasoconstriction and sodium and water retention.

There are a number of other factors that contribute to the formation of ascites, the main one being hypoalbuminaemia. This is associated with chronic liver disease, resulting in reduced plasma oncotic pressure and hence the leakage of plasma into the peritoneal cavity.

In most cases the onset of ascites is a sign of decompensated severe chronic liver disease and impaired liver function. However, it can also be present in non-liver conditions such as malnutrition, heart failure and nephrotic syndrome.

Gastro-oesophageal varices

Gastric and oesophageal varices are abnormally dilated collateral vessels in the stomach or oesophagus which arise as a result of increased portal vein pressure (portal hypertension) in cirrhosis or portal vein obstruction. The collateral vessels, or varices, enable blood to bypass

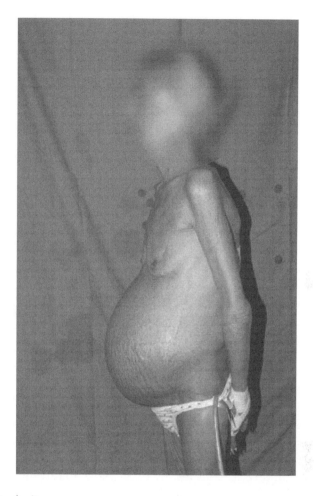

Figure 4.3 Ascites.

the liver or obstruction as a means of reducing the portal pressure. When the pressure in the vessels reaches a crucial point they can burst, leading to massive haemorrhage. This gastro-oesophageal bleeding is therefore associated with increased portal pressure, rather than acid erosion. Variceal bleeds are associated with high mortality, with up to 30% of first bleeds being fatal. Variceal bleeds are a sign of increased portal pressure, which is generally as a result of cirrhosis, although it can occur as a result of other conditions, such as Budd–Chiari syndrome (clotting in the hepatic vein leaving the liver). The presence of varices is suggestive of impaired liver function and reduced first-pass effect, as the portal blood may bypass the liver.

Hepatic encephalopathy

The term hepatic encephalopathy describes a spectrum of neuro-psychiatric changes that are usually reversible and which can occur with acute or chronic liver dysfunction. Hepatic encephalopathy is graded into four stages of increasing severity. In grade 1 the patient may be forgetful, confused and agitated, with sleep disturbances. In grade 2 they become increasingly disorientated and confused, with lethargy; by grade 4 the patient is unresponsive and in a coma. In hyperacute liver failure a patient will present within seven days with encephalopathy, which can be profound and may be accompanied by seizures. In chronic liver disease the signs can appear insidiously over months or more, quickly accompanying an episode of decompensating liver disease.

There are several theories behind the cause of hepatic encephalopathy. One of these is that the accumulation of toxins in the brain, particularly ammonia, is the cause. Ammonia is produced in the intestine and is usually metabolised in the liver to urea via the urea cycle. As a result of portosystemic shunting and reduced metabolism in the liver, ammonia serum levels rise as the transformation to urea is reduced. However, the validity of this theory is questionable as not all patients with signs of hepatic encephalopathy have raised serum ammonia levels. Another theory is that patients with hepatic encephalopathy have increased permeability of the blood–brain barrier, and hence the increased toxin levels permeate the brain more than usual, leading to altered neuropsychiatric function. There are also theories relating to increased levels of neurotransmitters, short-chain fatty acids, manganese and increased GABA-ergic transmission.

Hepatic encephalopathy is diagnosed by signs and symptoms. These include hepatic flap (which presents with hand tremor and an inability to keep the wrists extended on outstretched hands) and, in patients with subtle signs, several psychometric tests including 'serial 7s' and number connection tests. It is harder to diagnose in children, and so less specific signs, such as feeding difficulty and behavioural changes, are used.

The presence of hepatic encephalopathy suggests impaired liver function, the degree of impairment increasing with severity of encephalopathy. Any patient with encephalopathy will need careful consideration with regard to appropriate choice of drug and dosage.

Dupuytren's contracture

This is thickening of the tissue under the skin on the palms and fingers which causes the fingers to curl. It is common in patients with cirrhosis but can also occur in diabetics and epileptics. The cause is not known, although there is a genetic component, and in some cases it may be related to alcoholism. The presence of Dupuytren's contracture is not related to the degree of liver dysfunction.

Finger clubbing

This is an enlargement of the tips of the fingers and nails. It can also affect the toes. The cause is unknown, although theories include effects on dilatation of blood vessels and stimulation of various growth factors. Clubbing is common in advanced cirrhosis but is also present in lung, heart and other gastrointestinal diseases. The presence of clubbing does not give an indication of liver function.

Pruritus

Pruritus with no apparent dermatological cause can be a significant symptom in cholestatic liver conditions. It is thought to be associated with high concentrations of bile salts accumulating in the skin because they are not being excreted. There is also some suggestion that there is a central cause of the itch, as opiate receptor antagonists provide effective relief in some patients. It can occur all over the body, including the eyes and ears, but is usually most significant on the hands and feet.

Pruritus can have a significant impact on a patient's quality of life. The extent is very patient specific and does not indicate the degree of liver dysfunction; however, it can be the only indication for liver transplantation in patients with PBC and Alagille's syndrome, who have otherwise normal liver function.

Less specific signs and symptoms of liver dysfunction

Malnutitrition

Malnutrition is found in 80–100% of patients with decompensated liver disease, and in up to 40% of those with compensated disease. As the disease progresses patients become malnourished. Dry weight decreases, as they often reduce their food intake due to anorexia, malabsorption, nausea, vomiting and early satiety secondary to ascites. Inappropriate dietary restrictions can also be a cause of malnutrition.

In normal liver function, energy and protein requirements reduce as body mass reduces; however, cirrhotic patients can be hypermetabolic and therefore use calories and protein as if they had a higher body weight. If their intake is reduced, this exacerbates the weight loss. As the liver function deteriorates, a patient's malnutrition will worsen if not appropriately treated. Nutritional support is usually required to meet calorie and protein requirements. Malnutrition and associated symptoms are caused by many other conditions and are not specific to liver disease.

Peripheral oedema

Peripheral oedema is caused by fluid retention in the legs and ankles due to activation of the renin–angiotensin–aldosterone system. There are many causes of peripheral oedema other than liver dysfunction.

Bruising and bleeding

Patients with severe liver dysfunction are more prone to bruising and bleeding as a result of reduced clotting factor production or vitamin K deficiency. The severity increases with worsening liver function. Bruising and bleeding can also be caused by other coagulation disorders.

White nails

Leukonychia or white nails occur in chronic liver disease owing to the lack of albumin. It is not specific for liver disease and can also be present in renal failure, or may be congenital.

Splenomegaly

An enlargement of the spleen can be associated with many conditions, including infections, anaemias, malignancies and liver disease. In portal hypertension the back pressure in the splenic vein causes the spleen to enlarge.

Palmar erythema

This is a reddening of the palms of the hands and can affect the soles of the feet. It is associated with chronic liver disease but may also be present in a wide variety of conditions, such as pregnancy, rheumatoid arthritis and thyrotoxicosis. The cause is unknown, although it has been associated with high oestrogen levels.

Fatigue/malaise

Although not specific for liver dysfunction, patients with all types of liver disease often present with extreme fatigue and malaise. The fatigue generally worsens throughout the day. It is not a measure of extent of liver impairment, but can have a major effect on quality of life.

Right upper quadrant pain and abdominal pain

Right upper quadrant pain can be caused by stimulation of nerve endings in the liver capsule as a result of being stretched when the liver is enlarged or inflamed. It can also be as a result of gallbladder or colon problems. Ascites can cause abdominal pain as the tension of fluid in the abdominal cavity accumulates. The extent of the pain does not give an indication of liver function.

Muscle cramps

Many patients with severe liver disease suffer with muscle cramps, which are probably associated with electrolyte imbalances. They are non-specific for liver disease and do not give an indication of liver function.

Methods of grading overall liver function

Child–Pugh, MELD and PELD are three methodologies that have been developed to assess the severity of liver dysfunction.

Child–Pugh classification

This scoring system was originally developed in 1973 to determine the surgical risk of adult patients with bleeding varices. It takes into account the presence and degree of ascites and encephalopathy, serum albumin and bilirubin. Each of these parameters is weighted from 1 to 3. The sum of the scores gives a patient, at a specific point in time, a Child–Pugh classification of A, B or C. Classification A (score 5/6) is

Table 4.5 Scoring for Child–Pugh classification of severity of liver disease

Parameter/score	1	2	3
Ascites	None	Moderate or easily treated	Severe or intractable
Encephalopathy (grade)	None	1–2	3–4
Bilirubin (μmol/L)	<35	35–50	>50
Albumin (g/L)	>35	28–35	<28
INR	<1.7	1.8–2.3	>2.3

Child–Pugh A is a score of 5/6 (indicating a well-compensated liver).
Child–Pugh B is a score of 7–9 (indicating significant functional compromise).
Child–Pugh C is a score of 10–15 (indicating a decompensated liver).

considered well compensated disease, B (7–9) is significant functional compromise, and C (10–15) is decompensated disease. A patient's classification may increase or decrease over time, so regular reassessment is required (Table 4.5).

Model for end-stage liver disease (MELD) and paediatric end-stage liver disease (PELD)

MELD and PELD are scoring systems often used as a method of prioritising patients awaiting liver transplantation. Patients with a higher score are deemed to require a transplant more urgently than those with a lower score. The MELD system is for patients 12 years and older and PELD for those under 12.

Serum bilirubin, creatinine and INR are the parameters used to calculate a MELD score. For PELD, the calculation also takes into account growth failure and gives a higher weighting for children under one year. Scores can be as low as 6 for a well-compensated, low-priority patient, or as high as 60 for a severely ill patient. Scores may increase or decrease as the condition changes, so regular reassessment is needed.

Methods to quantify actual liver function

Several tests have been developed to quantify actual liver function, including indocyanine green (ICG), aminopyrine and bromosulphothalein. The principle of these tests is to determine whether hepatic blood flow or cell function is reduced by administering a chemical which is exclusively taken up or metabolised by the liver. For example, in the ICG clearance test the ICG is a non-toxic chemical solely taken up by the liver and eliminated unchanged. A dose is administered intravenously and plasma samples are taken at intervals to determine how quickly it is eliminated from the body. A lower result than normal suggests a reduced functional capacity of the liver.

In terms of the administration of medicines to patients with reduced liver function, the results of the above tests are of limited use. Even if it is known that there is a reduced blood flow to the liver it does not tell us how a patient will handle a particular medicine, and therefore these tests are usually more likely to be performed to give an indication of risk for a patient undergoing surgery.

Key points

- It is important to be able to determine which patients have a liver problem, and need to have their liver function taken into account when prescribing.
- There is no single method of determining liver function.
- The combination of trends in LFTs, other test results, diagnosis, and a patient's signs and symptoms need to be considered when assessing the degree of liver function.
- Abnormal LFTs do not necessarily indicate impaired liver function, as none is specific for the liver.
- A patient with a diseased liver may have normal LFTs.
- LFTs cannot be considered accurately without the clotting screen. It is the key method of determining functional capacity of the liver.

Guided further reading

Bircher J et al. (eds) (1999) *Oxford Textbook of Clinical Hepatology.* Oxford: Oxford Medical Publications.

Johnson PJ, MacFarlane IG. (1989) *The Laboratory Investigation of Liver Disease.* London: Baillière Tindall.

Laboratory Guidelines for Screening, Diagnosis and Monitoring of Hepatic Injury (2000) National Academy of Clinical Biochemistry (access via www.AASLD.org).

Sherlock S, Dooley J. (2001) *Diseases of the Liver and Biliary System.* Oxford: Blackwell Ltd.

Part Two

Principles of drug use in liver disease

5

Pharmacokinetics of drugs in liver disease

Trevor N Johnson and Alison H Thomson

Objectives

By the end of this chapter, the reader should be able to:

- Describe how liver disease may change the absorption, distribution, metabolism and excretion of medicines.
- Explain the differences between high extraction and low extraction ratio drugs.
- Describe the metabolic pathways that facilitate drug elimination from the body and list the ones that are most affected in liver disease.
- List the key biomarkers that indicate disease severity and may indicate the need for dose modification in liver disease.

Introduction

The pharmacokinetics of many drugs are altered in patients with liver disease. The clinical relevance of these changes depends on the elimination pathways for a particular drug and the nature and severity of the liver disease. In some conditions, such as schistosomiasis and viral hepatitis, impairment of drug elimination may not be sufficient to warrant a reduction of drug dosage, whereas in severe cirrhosis or some forms of carcinoma dosage adjustment may be necessary. The 'safe' use of drugs in hepatic disease requires an awareness of changes in both pharmacokinetics and pharmacodynamics.

Pharmacokinetics is the study of the relationships between the drug dosage regimen and the changes in drug concentration over time. Typically, concentrations are measured in blood, serum or plasma, and the concentration–time profile is described by a series of equations.

Knowledge of the relationships between drug concentrations in the blood and the clinical response (pharmacodynamics), which includes both therapeutic and toxic effects, is used to determine the concentration–time profile that is likely to be associated with optimal response and minimum risk of toxicity. In patients with altered pharmacokinetic parameters, drug dosage regimens may need to be changed to ensure that concentration–time profiles remain optimal. These adjustments typically involve changes in dose amount, dosage interval or both.

Hepatic disease and drug pharmacokinetics

Biochemical criteria ('liver function tests') and clotting time are often used to assess the degree of liver dysfunction. However, unlike renal disease, in which creatinine concentration can be used to predict drug clearance, there is no biochemical or haematological measurement that determines the extent to which hepatic disease will affect the clearance of a specific drug. For example, elevation of the hepatic enzymes aspartate aminotransferase (AST) and alanine aminotransferase (ALT) indicates liver damage, whereas low concentrations of protein and albumin can indicate a reduction in the synthetic capacity of the liver. None of these measurements directly reflects the metabolic function of the liver. In addition, variations in effect can depend on the type of illness: for example, acute viral hepatitis may have little effect on drug clearance, whereas the impact of chronic hepatitis is likely to depend on the degree of cirrhosis. The characteristics of the drug, such as its 'extraction ratio', the metabolic pathways involved and the extent of biliary secretion are also important; therefore, different drugs can be affected in different ways under different clinical circumstances.

Comparisons of drug pharmacokinetics in hepatic disease have often been based on classifications of mild, moderate or severe disease, e.g. the Child–Pugh score [1, 2], but such categories were developed to predict disease outcome rather than drug handling. An investigation into this problem conducted by the Swedish Regulatory Agency [3] suggested that serum albumin is the best overall predictor of drug handling, and that prothrombin time and bilirubin may also be useful. Indeed, serum bilirubin cut-offs for dose reduction (in liver disease, not cholestasis) are quoted in the SPC (Summary of Product Characteristics) for epirubicin, but a study has shown that bilirubin was a poor predictor of epirubicin clearance [4]. The reduced clearance of some anticancer drugs has been associated with elevated AST and ALT concentrations. For example, a study of epirubicin pharmacokinetics in patients with advanced breast cancer, many of whom had liver metastases [4], found that AST was a more reliable indicator of epirubicin clearance than bilirubin and dosage guidelines based on this measurement were developed.

Pharmacokinetic principles

There are three fundamental processes that determine drug dosage regimens: absorption, distribution and elimination. Three pharmacokinetic parameters are associated with these processes: bioavailability (absorption), volume of distribution (distribution and elimination) and clearance (elimination).

Absorption

Bioavailability is defined as the extent – and sometimes also the rate – of drug absorption. For oral therapy, absolute bioavailability is usually determined by comparing the area under the concentration–time curve (AUC) after an oral dose with that after an intravenous dose. Assuming clearance is constant, bioavailability is defined as the ratio of oral to intravenous AUC, corrected for dose, and is expressed as a proportion or a percentage. For example, an oral bioavailability of around 20% means that an oral dose of 100 mg would achieve an exposure equivalent to that of an intravenous dose of 20 mg. For some drugs with low bioavailability due to a high first-pass metabolism, oral dose requirements may be lower in patients with severe hepatic disease due to a reduction in first-pass metabolism in the liver and consequent increase in bioavailability [1]. In contrast, reduced bioavailability of lipophilic drugs may occur in cholestasis and has been reported with ciclosporin, particularly with early formulations [5].

Distribution

Once the drug is absorbed into the systemic circulation, the extent of its distribution to the tissues depends on a range of factors, including lipid solubility, plasma protein binding and tissue binding. The apparent 'volume of distribution' reflects the relationship between the amount of drug in the body and the concentration that can be measured in the plasma or serum. For example, if a drug is very water soluble with little plasma protein binding, the volume of distribution often reflects the volume of the extracellular fluid (around 0.25 L/kg body weight). In contrast, if a drug is very lipid soluble or highly bound in the tissues, the concentration of drug in the serum will be low and the apparent volume will be high. Drugs that bind strongly to plasma proteins may have a relatively low volume of distribution (e.g. warfarin, which is 99% bound, has a volume of distribution of 0.14 L/kg), but lipid solubility and tissue binding are also important (e.g. diazepam, which is also 99% bound, has a volume of distribution of 1.1 L/kg). Loading doses of drugs are usually based on the volume of distribution, the aim being to 'fill up' the volume with sufficient drug to achieve a target drug concentration quickly, as presented in Panel 5.1.

Panel 5.1 Basic pharmacokinetic terms and relationships

Volume of distribution (V) is the apparent volume that relates the amount of drug in the body (A) to the measured concentration (C). It is often used to calculate a loading dose.

Loading dose = Target C $\times$ V

Clearance (CL) is the volume of blood, plasma or serum cleared of drug per unit time. It relates the dosing rate to the average steady-state concentration (Css_{av}) and is used to calculate the maintenance dose of a drug.

Maintenance dose rate = Target $Css_{av} \times$ CL

Elimination rate constant (k) determines the rate of decline of a concentration and the rate of accumulation to steady state. It depends on CL and V.

k = CL/V

Elimination half-life ($t_{1/2}$) is the time taken for the concentration to fall to half. In five half-lives 97% of a dose would be eliminated and 97% of steady state would be achieved on multiple dosing. It depends on CL and V.

$(t_{1/2}) = -\,Ln(0.5)/k = 0.693\ V/CL$

In hepatic disease, changes in plasma protein binding, tissue binding and fluid balance can occur that might influence the apparent volume of distribution. Albumin is responsible for most binding of drugs in plasma, particularly acidic and neutral compounds such as ibuprofen, valproic acid, phenytoin and prednisolone. Many basic drugs, such as methadone and verapamil, bind to both albumin and α_1-acid glycoprotein (an acute-phase reactant that is often released in response to stress) [6]. Low albumin and α_1-acid glycoprotein concentrations arising from a reduction in synthesis, changes in albumin binding affinity due to conformational changes in the molecule, and the accumulation of endogenous substances such as bilirubin, are features of chronic liver disease that can lead to a reduction in plasma protein binding and increase in free fraction [6].

A reduction in albumin binding would lead to a fall in the bound and hence the total concentrations of drug in the plasma, but the unbound concentration would usually be unchanged. For example, a total phenytoin concentration of 15 mg/L in a patient with an albumin concentration of 30 g/L would be equivalent to a total concentration of 21 mg/L if the albumin concentration had been normal. This can be seen by applying a commonly used equation for correcting phenytoin concentrations in hypoalbuminaemia [7], i.e.

$$\text{Corrected concentration} = \frac{\text{Measured concentration}}{(0.9 \times \text{albumin}/44) + 0.1} \qquad \text{(Eqn 5.1)}$$

This assumes that with 'normal' albumin concentrations (taken as 44 g/L in this example) phenytoin is 90% bound and 10% unbound. A further correction to this equation has been proposed to account for reduced binding in renal failure, but there is no equivalent for hepatic disease, although changes in binding have been reported in viral hepatitis [8].

As bound concentration falls, the free concentration is more available for distribution and elimination, and as total concentrations are therefore lower, hypoalbuminaemia can lead to an increase in apparent volume of distribution. However, tissue distribution may also change in hepatic disease. This is illustrated by tolbutamide in viral hepatitis. No change was found in the volume of distribution of tolbutamide because changes in plasma protein binding were matched by changes in tissue binding [9].

Other features of severe hepatic disease include elevation of plasma volume and ascites (accumulation of fluid in the peritoneal cavity), leading to an increase in the volumes of distribution of water-soluble drugs, such as the aminoglycoside antibiotics. Because elimination half-life depends on clearance and volume of distribution, this increase will result in a longer elimination half-life. In such cases, higher doses with longer intervals may be required to maintain target concentrations (a high peak and a low trough).

Elimination

The efficiency of drug elimination from the body depends on clearance, which in turn depends on body function. For drugs cleared principally by renal excretion, kidney function determines the efficiency of elimination, whereas for drugs that are mainly cleared by hepatic metabolism, liver blood flow, access to hepatic enzymes and enzyme function are the defining factors. As clearance determines the relationship between dosing rate and average steady-state concentration (Panel 5.1), changes in clearance can lead to changes in the maintenance dose requirements of drugs.

Clearance reflects the volume of fluid cleared per time, whereas the rate of drug elimination from the body, as described by the elimination rate constant k, depends on both clearance and volume of distribution. A related parameter, the elimination half-life, which is the time it takes for the concentration to fall to half, also depends on both clearance and volume of distribution. These relationships are summarised in Panel 5.1. Changes in clearance or volume of distribution that lead to an increase in elimination half-life will prolong the time it takes for a drug to be eliminated from the body, which may allow the dosage interval to be increased, e.g. from 12 hours to 24 hours.

Hepatic clearance

Drug clearance is often defined as the product of blood flow (delivery of drug to the organ of removal) and extraction ratio (the proportion of the drug concentration that is removed as the drug passes through the organ). Extraction ratio (ER) can be defined as follows:

$$ER = Cin - Cout/Cin \qquad\qquad (Eqn\ 5.2)$$

where Cin represents the concentration entering the liver and Cout the concentration leaving the liver. ER can therefore range from 0 (no extraction) to 1 (complete extraction) and represents the efficiency of drug removal by the liver.

It has been demonstrated that hepatic extraction ratio (ER) is also influenced by blood flow. A number of mathematical models have been proposed to explain this observation, but the simplest model, and the one that is easiest to apply to clinical practice, is the 'well stirred' or 'venous equilibrium' model (Equation 5.3). This model relates hepatic clearance to hepatic blood flow (Q), the fraction of drug concentration that is unbound in plasma (fu) and the intrinsic clearance of the unbound drug (Cl_uint) [1]. Intrinsic clearance represents the maximum clearance of drug in the absence of any restrictions caused by blood flow, binding or access to the metabolising enzymes. The model states that:

Hepatic

clearance $(L/h) = Q (L/h) \times ER = Q (L/h) \times \dfrac{fu. Cl_uint}{Q + fu. Cl_uint}$ (Eqn 5.3)

This model has been used to predict what might happen to drug handling and dose requirements under different clinical circumstances by categorising drugs according to their extraction ratio [1].

High extraction ratio drugs (ER >0.7)

Absorption

When a drug that is eliminated mainly by metabolism in the liver is administered orally, it is delivered first to the liver, where it can be metabolised on 'first pass'. Assuming complete absorption, and in the absence of metabolism in the intestinal wall, bioavailability can be estimated from 1 – extraction ratio. In the absence of portosystemic shunts, a fall in blood flow through the liver could potentially reduce bioavailability, as the slower flow offers more opportunity for metabolism to occur. However, if the extraction ratio is reduced, e.g. due to a decrease in intrinsic clearance, or the development of shunts that enable blood to bypass functioning hepatocytes, both of which can occur in severe cirrhosis, bioavailability will increase and the dose may have to be reduced. For example, morphine, which has an extraction ratio of about 0.7, has an oral bioavailability of around 30% in healthy individuals but around 100% in patients with severe cirrhosis [10]. Changes in extraction ratio due to hepatic disease can therefore have a clinically significant effect on the bioavailability of a high extraction ratio drug.

Elimination

When the extraction ratio is high, clearance is so efficient that fu. Cl_uint dominates the denominator of the hepatic clearance model and Q becomes negligible. As fu. Cl_uint then cancels out, hepatic blood flow becomes the most important factor influencing drug elimination (Panel 6.2), and changes to fraction unbound or intrinsic clearance are less important.

Hepatic clearance $= Q \times \dfrac{\cancel{fu. Cl_uint}}{Q + \cancel{fu. Cl_uint}} \approx Q$

However, in severe hepatic disease, not only is hepatic blood flow reduced but the degree of liver damage may influence intrinsic clearance to the extent that it also affects total drug clearance. Consequently, patients with hepatic disease are at particular risk of developing adverse effects to high extraction ratio drugs.

The consequences of changes in protein binding to the pharmacokinetics of high extraction drugs are complex. In normal circumstances, the reliance of total drug clearance on hepatic blood flow means that total drug concentrations are unlikely to be affected by reductions in protein binding, and so the unbound concentration may increase, giving rise to misinterpretation of the (unchanged) total concentration and potential toxicity. Dose adjustments due to changes in drug handling may therefore be necessary. However, the outcome may be different in severe hepatic disease if intrinsic clearance falls to the extent that the drug develops 'intermediate' extraction ratio properties. If this happens, application of the full equation indicates that both total and unbound concentrations may be altered because the drug elimination becomes less 'flow dependent' and more dependent on a combination of blood flow, intrinsic clearance and fraction unbound. These complex relationships can make it difficult to predict how drug concentrations and dosage requirements might be altered.

Low extraction ratio drugs (<0.3)

Absorption

For drugs with a low extraction ratio, oral bioavailability is typically high, as most of the dose will be unaffected by the liver on first pass. Consequently, changes in extraction ratio are unimportant. For example, if hepatic disease caused a fall in extraction ratio from 0.1 to 0.05, bioavailability would only increase from 90% to 95%, which is unlikely to be clinically significant.

Elimination

For drugs with a low extraction ratio, Q is much greater than fu. Cl_uint, therefore fu. Cl_uint has a minimal effect on the denominator. The clearance model can therefore be simplified as follows:

$$\text{Hepatic clearance} = \cancel{Q} \times \frac{\text{fu. } Cl_u\text{int}}{\cancel{Q} + \text{fu. } Cl_u\text{int}} \approx \text{fu. } Cl_u\text{int}$$

As clearance of total drug mainly depends on fu and Cl_uint, anything that influences enzyme function, such as enzyme inducers or inhibitors, or severe hepatic disease, will potentially have a clinically significant influence on drug clearance and dosage requirements. Low extraction ratio drugs can be further divided according to the degree of plasma protein binding. When binding is low, changes in fraction unbound will have little impact on clearance, but when plasma protein binding is high relative to the extraction ratio (e.g. fu < 20%, or % bound > 80%) an increase in fu will lead to a fall in total drug concentration and an increase in total drug clearance, as illustrated in Panel 5.2. However, unbound (active) drug concentrations should not change, and therefore dose requirements will be unaltered. Displacement interactions, such as displacement of phenytoin by tolbutamide or salicylate, have a similar effect [6]. In contrast, if both protein binding and intrinsic clearance are reduced by the interacting drug, such as occurs with valproic acid and phenytoin, a reduction in phenytoin dose might be required, as both free fraction and free concentration would increase. Similar requirements to reduce dose would occur in liver disease if both hepatic metabolism and protein binding were affected.

In patients with hepatic disease there are a number of competing factors that make predictions of clinical outcome difficult. For example, the extent to which drug metabolism is altered is difficult to assess, as it is often only in severe hepatic disease that certain metabolic pathways are affected. Although protein binding changes are often thought to be important, with the possible exception of highly bound (> 80%) high extraction ratio (> 0.7) drugs, changes in dose requirements generally only occur when metabolic capacity is reduced. Otherwise, the main concern is potential misinterpretation of total drug concentration measurements.

Panel 5.2 summarises the predictions of the well-stirred model for low and high extraction ratio drugs. For low extraction ratio drugs, insignificant changes in bioavailability occur with changes in blood flow, fraction unbound or intrinsic clearance, whereas all three can significantly influence the bioavailability of high extraction ratio drugs. In contrast, the model suggests that total clearance of high extraction ratio drugs is only altered by blood flow, whereas both fraction unbound and intrinsic clearance affect the clearance of low extraction ratio drugs. It must be remembered, however, that if the drug is highly protein bound, the total concentration measurement may be misleading. Ideally, unbound concentration should be measured for all highly protein bound drugs, but this is technically more difficult and therefore not routine practice.

Panel 5.2 Summary of the predictions of the well-stirred model of hepatic clearance (based on total drug concentration)

	Changes			Consequences	
	Blood flow	fu	Cl_{int}	CL	F
Low	↓ –	–	–	–	–
extraction	–	↑	–	↑	–
	–	–	↓	↓	–
High	↓ –	–	–	↓ –	↓
extraction	–	↑	–	–	↓
	–	–	↓		↑

Intermediate extraction ratio drugs (0.3–0.7)

Although most drugs are can be categorised as high or low extraction, some can be defined as 'intermediate' extraction. In addition, the influence of hepatic disease, if severe, may change a high extraction ratio drug into the 'intermediate' category. For such drugs, and particularly in severe cirrhosis, where protein binding, intrinsic clearance and hepatic blood flow may all be altered, it is difficult to predict the clinical outcomes. Furthermore, the well-stirred model is an oversimplification that does not adequately explain the handling of all drugs, even in patients with normal hepatic function.

Biliary excretion

Some drugs, such as digoxin, doxorubicin, paclitaxel, morphine, and many drug metabolites, particularly glucuronides, glutathione and sulphate conjugates, are actively secreted into bile by a range of protein transporters, including P-glycoprotein (MDR1) and MRP2 [1]. Cholestasis, in which bile formation or flow is reduced, leads to the accumulation of bile in the liver, injury to the hepatocytes and, in advanced cases of biliary cirrhosis, a reduction in intrinsic clearance. In addition, restriction to biliary flow will reduce 'enterohepatic recycling' in which breakdown of the metabolite by endogenous gut bacteria leads to regeneration of the parent drug, which can be reabsorbed. This will effectively reduce the patient's exposure to the drug through the recycling mechanism.

Drug metabolism in liver disease

Overview of drug metabolism

Drug metabolism is normally divided into two phases, phase 1 or functionalisation reactions, and phase 2 conjugation reactions. Phase 1 reactions produce or uncover a chemical reactive group on which the phase 2 reactions can occur. The phase 2 reaction is usually the true detoxification pathway, resulting in water-soluble products that are easily excreted. The cytochrome P450 system that catalyses the mixed-function oxidation of xenobiotics comprises the most important group of enzymes involved in phase 1 metabolism; others include the flavin-containing mono-oxygenases. The common phase 2 or conjugation reactions include glucuronidation, glycosidation, sulphation, methylation, acetylation and glutathione conjugation.

The CYP are a growing superfamily of around 500 enzymes spread across different species, grouped according to their amino acid sequence [11]. A homology greater than 40% defines a family, and greater than 55% defines a subfamily. The symbol CYP is used to denote both human and rat cytochrome P450 (cyp is used for mouse and drosophila). CYP is followed by an Arabic numeral denoting the family, a capital letter designating the subfamily, and then another Arabic numeral representing the individual gene or enzyme. An example would be:

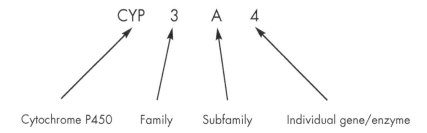

CYP enzymes in human liver

Seven isoforms account for the total CYP protein mass found in human liver [12]. These are summarised in Figure 5.1.

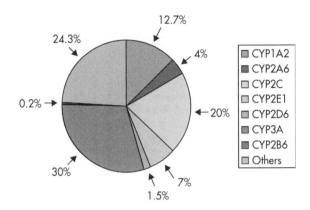

Figure 5.1 Major CYP enzymes expressed in human liver. Amounts are expressed as a percentage of total CYP protein.

Five CYP subfamilies appear to be principally involved in hepatic drug metabolism, namely CYPs 1A, 2C, 2D, 2E and 3A. Within these groups the specific isoforms of importance are CYPs 1A2, 2C8–10, 2C19, 2D6, 2E1, 3A4 and 3A5. CYPs 2A6 and 2B6 were thought to play a minor role, but their significance is becoming more apparent. CYP3A4 is the most important CYP, as it is involved in the metabolism of 50% of currently used drugs [13].

Measurement of CYP enzyme expression and activity

In vivo

In vivo probe substrates are available to assess the activity of particular enzymes, for example midazolam for CYP3A4/5, caffeine for CYP1A2 and tolbutamide for CYP2C9 [14].

In vitro

Microsomes are closed vesicles of fragments of the endoplasmic reticular membrane and contain several drug-metabolising enzymes, including CYPs. Enzyme expression and activity can be measured in microsomes. Immunoblotting using specific monoclonal antibodies is often employed to assess the expression of CYP enzymes, and specific drug probes (and cofactors) can be incubated with the microsomes to gain knowledge of the *in vitro* activity. *In vitro* drug probes include testosterone and midazolam for CYP3A, S-mephenytoin for CYPs 2B6 and 2C19, and ethoxyresorufin for CYP1A2 [15].

Age-dependent changes in hepatic drug elimination

The individual drug-metabolising enzymes follow different developmental patterns. An indication of when the various enzymes are first expressed is given below:

- Expression in foetal liver with activity towards endogenous compounds, e.g. CYP3A7 [15, 16], sulphotransferase [17]. In the case of CYP3A7 expression declines rapidly after birth, to be replaced by CYP3A4/5. Sulphotransferase activity continues.
- Expression in the early neonatal period within hours after birth but with minimal expression in the foetal liver, e.g. CYP2D6 [18], CYP2E1 [19] and glucuronidation [20].
- Expression later in neonatal development, e.g. CYP1A2 [21], CYP3A4 [15, 16].

The developmental patterns of both phase 1 and phase 2 enzymes have been extensively reviewed [22, 23].

Phase 1 enzymes

Because of the low expression of many of the CYP enzymes in the first month of life the hepatic clearance of many drugs is reduced. Examples include the prolonged half-life of phenytoin in preterm infants (~75 h) compared to term infants (~20h) [24], and the reduced weight normalised clearance of midazolam in preterm (0.072–0.096 L/kg/h) compared to term neonates (0.11–0.13 L/kg/h) [25]. Metabolic clearance then increases to a maximum by between two and ten years of age, followed by a steady decline into adulthood. In a study by Hughes *et al.* midazolam clearance was higher in children aged three to 13 years (0.78 L/kg/h) than in adults (0.38–0.66 L/kg/h) [26]. There are many examples of hepatically metabolised drugs that exhibit a higher systemic weight normalised clearance in children than in adults, including theophylline [27], phenytoin [28] and carbamazepine [29]. Possible reasons for increased weight normalised clearance in young children are increased concentrations of catalytically active CYPs per unit of liver or an increased liver volume normalised to body size. Evidence to date would indicate that increased relative liver size is the most likely explanation [30, 31].

Phase 2 enzymes

At birth, compounds that rely on glucuronidation for elimination have prolonged half-lives compared to those in adults. Morphine clearance is five times lower in neonates (two to 12 days) than in children aged one to 16 years. Morphine is cleared faster in children over one than in adults [32].

In general, the foetus expresses significant sulphotransferase activity [20]. For some drugs that undergo extensive glucuronidation in adults, sulphation may become the predominant pathway. Sulphation may play a larger role in the metabolism of paracetamol in children than in adults. The ratio of glucuronide to sulphate is around 2 in adults, 0.8 in children aged three to ten, and 0.35 in neonates [33, 34].

For children with liver disease, developmental changes have to be considered in parallel with the effects of the disease when determining the optimal dose of a drug.

Altered drug metabolism in liver disease

Drug metabolism is impaired in patients with liver disease, with CYP-mediated reactions affected more than phase 2 enzymes [35]. Impairment of CYP expression and activity correlates with the severity of liver disease and also, for some of the enzymes, the aetiology of cirrhosis.

Phase 1 enzymes

The effects of liver disease on the phase 1 enzymes have recently been reviewed [36, 37].

Cytochrome P450

In animals and humans with cholestatic and non-cholestatic cirrhosis the total expression and activity of CYP enzymes is equally reduced, by around 48% [38], and were significantly less than in controls. This reduction is not uniform: CYPs 1A, 2C19 and 3A appear to be particularly sensitive to the effects of liver disease, whereas with CYPs 2A, 2D6, 2C9 and 2E1 this is less so. A comprehensive review of the literature on alteration of CYP enzymes in liver cirrhosis is given in Table 5.1.

Table 5.1 Changes in the individual human CYP enzymes in cirrhosis

CYP	Reduction in expression (in vitro)	Reduction in activity (in vitro)	Drugs clearance reduced (in vivo)	Comments	References
CYP1A2	30%–53% ↓ in CYP1A expression	↓ O-dealkylation of ethoxyresorufin in cirrhosis	Caffeine Theophylline Antipyrine	Decrease in expression greater in cirrhosis without cholestasis	[38–43]
CYP2A6			↓ in patients with moderate/severe disease	CYP2A6 activity measured by urinary excretion of 7-hydroxycoumarin	[44]
CYP2B		Reduced ECOD in PBC		Measured in human liver microsomes	[45]
CYP2B		↔ 7-ethoxycoumarin metabolism in PBC & controls		Measured in human liver microsomes	[46]
CYP2C	↔ protein levels compared to controls up to 68% and 41% ↓ in CYP2C protein				[38]
CYP2C				Measured in human microsomes from cholestatic and non-cholestatic cirrhosis, respectively	[39]
CYP2C19			↓ CL of omeprazole S-mephenytoin Aminopyrine	CYP2C19 thought to be very sensitive to even mild cirrhosis	[47–50]
CYP2C9		↔ hydroxylation of tolbutamide	Clearance of tolbutamide normal in cirrhosis		[51]

(continued)

Table 5.1 Continued

CYP	Reduction in expression (in vitro)	Reduction in activity (in vitro)	Drugs clearance reduced (in vivo)	Comments	References
CYP2C9 & CYP2C19			Mephenytoin Urinary excretion of 4-hydroxymephenytoin from S isomer ↓ by 28% in mild and 62% in moderate liver disease	Mephenytoin is a standard *in vivo* probe, the R isomer metabolized by CYP2C9 and the S isomer by CYP2C19	[52]
CYP2C8	↔ in CYP2C8			End-stage liver disease	[53]
CYP2C9	CYP2C9 ↓ in small number of cases			End-stage liver disease	[53]
CYP2D6			Conflicting evidence ↔ in debrisoquine clearance		[52]
CYP2D6			Propafenone CL ↓ by 40%		[54]
CYP2E1	↔ or ↓			Effect may depend on aetiology of cirrhosis- only subjects with severe cholestatic liver disease have reduction in CYP2E1. Another confounding factor is effects of alcohol	[38, 39, 53]
CYP3A	↓	↓6β-hydroxytestosterone hydroxylase activity ↓ erythromycin N-demethylation		CYP3A protein expression and activity ↓ in cirrhosis	[38, 39, 55]

Table 5.1 Continued

CYP	Reduction in expression (in vitro)	Reduction in activity (in vitro)	Drugs clearance reduced (in vivo)	Comments	References
CYP3A4			↓ CL of nifedipine		[56]
CYP3A4			↓ Lidocaine metabolism to MEGX	Plasma concentrations of MEGX severe cirrhosis = 4.6 ng/mL moderate cirrhosis = 19.1 ng/mL mild cirrhosis = 32.8 ng/mL control = 53.4 ng/mL Hence the more severe the cirrhosis the lower the metabolism of lidocaine to MEGX due to ↓ CYP3A4	[44]
CYP3A4			Twofold ↓ in midazolam CL 2.4-fold ↓ in midazolam $t_{1/2}$		[57–59]
CYP3A4			Twofold ↓ in CL of verapamil, isradipine, nitrendipine and nifedipine		[56, 60–62]
CYP3A4		↔ ethylmorphine demethylation			[63]
CYP3A4	↔ protein				[53]

As CYP2E1 is induced by alcohol, a patient with cirrhosis caused by chronic alcohol ingestion may express increased or unaltered levels of the enzyme whereas other cirrhotic patients may express reduced levels.
ECOD = ethoxycoumarin O-demethylation, a non-specific marker of CYP2B; PBC = primary biliary cirrhosis; MEGX = monoethylglycinexylide.

Severity of liver disease
In humans the elimination of several *in vivo* CYP probe drugs has been shown to correlate with the severity of cirrhosis, including aminopyrine [48, 50], lidocaine [64], caffeine [65], mephenytoin [47, 52] and antipyrine [66, 67]. In a study by Frye *et al.* [68] the metabolic clearance of four probe substrates (caffeine, CYP1A2; mephenytoin, CYP2C19; debrisoquine, CYP2D6; and chlorzoxazone, CYP2E1) was measured in 20 patients with different severity of liver disease and in 20 matched controls. In all cases there was a strong correlation between the Child–Pugh score and the extent of hepatic metabolism.

Type of liver disease
A number of the CYP enzymes change according to the type of cirrhosis (Table 5.1). Hasler *et al.* reported the percentage change in CYP1A2, 2C, 2E1 and 3A protein expression compared to controls for hepatocellular and cholestatic cirrhosis [13]. The results are shown in Table 5.2.

Table 5.2 Effects of different types of liver disease on the percentage reduction in normal expressed levels of individual P450 proteins

Type of cirrhosis	CYP1A2	CYP2C	CYP2E1	CYP3A
Hepatocellular	29	57	81	25
Cholestatic	18	34	49	41

Effects of liver transplantation on CYPs
By one year post liver transplant both CYP expression and activity are similar to those of normal subjects [67]. Some interesting effects are observed in the first six months after transplant, but some may be due to the induction of specific enzymes by therapeutic agents used in this period. The observation of a tenfold increase in hepatic CYP3A4 content at ten days which then returns to normal at six months is probably due to the administration of prednisolone in the early postoperative period [69]. Other observations are more difficult to explain. An eightfold increase in CYP2E1 as measured by the chlorzoxazone metabolic ratio has been detected in the first month post transplant [70]. CYP2E1-mediated NAPQI formation from paracetamol is also increased by around 137% and 81% on days two and ten post transplant, and returns to normal after six months [71].

Other phase 1 enzymes

There is a general lack of information on the effects of liver disease on other phase 1 enzymes, especially flavin-containing mono-oxygenases and monoamine oxidases (MAO). Indirect evidence suggests that hepatic MAO may be reduced in liver disease. MAO plays a dominant role in the metabolism of the triptan class of anti-migraine drugs, and MAO-A is the principal enzyme responsible for the clearance of sumatriptan and almotriptan [72, 73]. Therefore, patients with liver disease may be exposed to higher drug concentrations than those with normal hepatic function. Xanthine oxidase (XO) is involved in the conversion of 1-methylxanthine, a secondary metabolite of caffeine, to 1-methyluric acid. A slight increase in serum XO has been observed in two studies in patients with cirrhosis [74, 75]. In another study, there was no observed difference in XO serum concentration or activity between patients with cirrhosis and controls [76].

Alcohol dehydrogenase (ADH) is involved in the metabolism of ethanol to acetaldehyde, which in turn is converted to acetate by aldehyde dehydrogenase (ALDH). Because the hepatic expressions of these enzymes are influenced by both ethanol consumption and liver cirrhosis, which may be the consequence of ethanol consumption, it is sometimes difficult to know which of these factors is resulting in modulation of the enzyme. There is generally a reduction in ADH in alcoholic cirrhosis [77, 78], whereas in non-alcoholic cirrhotic patients some studies have detected a reduction in ADH [77] but others have detected no change [78]. Total ALDH is reduced in primary biliary cirrhosis, alcoholic and non-alcoholic cirrhosis compared to controls [77, 78].

Phase 2 enzymes

The effects of liver cirrhosis on the phase 2 enzymes has recently been reviewed by Elbekai *et al.* [36].

Glucuronidation

Glucuronidation is an important detoxification pathway in humans. Many therapeutic drugs and their metabolites are substrates for UDP-glucuronyltransferase (UGT), leading to the formation of usually inactive glucuronides, which are then excreted via bile or urine. Individual UGT enzymes are defined in a similar way to the CYP enzymes by family (1 or 2), subfamily (A or B) and an Arabic numeral representing the individual gene product. The important human UGTs are 1A1, 1A3, 1A4, 1A6, 1A9, 1A10, 2B4, 2B7, 2B15 and 2B17.

There was some early evidence that glucuronidation may be spared in liver cirrhosis. In a study using ethinyloestradiol, an *in vivo* probe for UGT1A1, and 1-napthol, an *in vivo* probe for UGT1A6, neither of these enzymes was found to be significantly altered in cirrhosis compared to controls [79]. Theories have been put forward as to why glucuronidation may be spared, including:

- An increase in UGT expression in remaining viable liver cells [80].
- Induction of extra hepatic glucuronidation, e.g. an apparent increased morphine extrahepatic glucuronidation in liver disease, possibly in the kidney, and to a lesser extent in the intestine [81].
- Most of the studies were in subjects with mild or moderate liver disease.

There is now much wider evidence to suggest that glucuronidation involving certain specific isoforms of the UGT enzyme is impaired in severe liver disease. The *in vitro* glucuronidation of zidovudine by UGT2B7 is significantly decreased in liver cirrhosis [82]. By contrast, glucuronidation of oxazepam and lamotrigine by UGT1A3 and 1A4 respectively remained unchanged [82]. However, the plasma half-life of lorazepam was increased in liver cirrhosis [83]. In patients with liver cirrhosis the ratio of unconjugated to conjugated paracetamol was increased [84]. Liver disease would appear to have variable effects on specific isoforms of the enzyme.

Sulphation

Sulphation is a major conjugation pathway in humans. The activity of sulphotransferase (SULT) towards 2-napthol has been shown to be significantly reduced in biopsy samples from patients with cirrhosis and chronic active hepatitis [79]. In another study sulphotransferase activities were decreased significantly in cirrhosis compared to the control group [85]. More recently, the activity of dehydroepiandrosterone sulphotransferase, a measure of SULT2A/2B activity, has been shown to be reduced in patients with primary biliary cirrhosis and alcoholic cirrhosis [86].

Acetyltransferase

The activity of acetyltransferase as measured by the rate of acetylation of p-aminobenzoic acid was significantly reduced in liver biopsy samples from subjects with cirrhosis compared to controls [79].

Glutathione S-transferase

GSTs are cytosolic enzymes that play a major role in the protection against chemical toxins and carcinogens. In human studies serum GST activities in liver cirrhosis were not significantly different from those of healthy controls [87], although GST activity towards benzo(a)pyrene-4,5 oxide was significantly reduced in liver biopsy samples from subjects with cirrhosis compared to controls.

Liver disease and hepatic blood flow

Total hepatic blood flow is often unchanged in patients with cirrhosis [88]; however, confounding underlying mechanisms often contribute to this observation. In patients with portal hypertension caused by cirrhosis there is often a reduction in portal venous flow and a compensatory increase in hepatic arterial blood flow [89, 90]. Many cirrhotic patients develop portal bypass, a condition in which a significant fraction of portal blood bypasses parenchymal tissue in the liver or enters directly into the superior vena cava via oesophageal varices. The presence of portal shunts coupled with reduced hepatic metabolism can greatly increase the oral bioavailability of drugs that undergo extensive first-pass metabolism. A greater than twofold increase in propranolol bioavailability has been shown in patients with cirrhosis compared to healthy controls [91].

Transjugular intrahepatic portosystemic shunt (TIPS) is a side-to-side non-selective portosystemic shunt that is frequently performed in cirrhosis to manage the complications of portal hypertension, such as variceal bleeding. The observation that the bioavailability of oral midazolam was significantly higher in cirrhotic patients with TIPS than in cirrhotic controls and healthy volunteers [57] may be due to reduced intestinal CYP3A activity or reduced contact with CYP3A in the enterocyte due to increased splanchnic blood flow [57, 92].

Effects of liver disease on the pharmacokinetics of hepatically cleared drugs

A summary of the effects of liver cirrhosis and its severity on the metabolism and pharmacokinetic parameters of selected drugs is shown in Table 5.3.

Table 5.3 Summary of selected *in vivo* studies investigating the effects of liver cirrhosis on the pharmacokinetics of drugs

Drug	Metabolism	Child–Pugh class (n)	PK observation						Study recommendations	References
			CL (L/h)	AUC (ng/mL/h) (μg/mL/h)*	$T_{1/2}$ (h)	C_{Max} (ng/mL)	T_{Max} (h)			
Amprenavir	CYP3A4	Control (10)	56	12	5.6	4.9	1	450 mg bd – moderate	[93]
		A/B (10)	34	26	7.8	6.5	1	300 mg bd – severe	
		C (10)	18	39	7.9	9.4	1		
Atomoxetine	CYP2D6	Control (10)	41	710	4	142	1	↓ dose 50% moderate	[94]
		B (6)	20	1200	11	115	3	↓ dose 75% severe	
		C (4)	11	2700	16	126	6		
Budesonide	CYP3A	A (12)	600	5.1	2.3	1.5	4.8	Not recommended in late stage PBC	[95]
		C (7)	410	23	5.8	4.9	5.0		
Clarithromycin	CYP3A4	Control (5)		3600				No dosage adjustments necessary	[83]
		A/B (7)		4970					
		C (6)		3200					
Clopidogrel	CYP3A4/5	Control (12)		6.3		2.6	1	No dosage adjustments needed in class A or B	[96]
		A/B (12)		8.2		2.4	1		
Doxazosin		Control (12)	12.8	172	22	12.3	3	No dose adjustments in mild/moderate cirrhosis	[97]
		A (12)	8.9	246	24	10.8	4		
Esomeprazole	CYP2C19/ 3A4	Control (36)		4.71*	1.5	1731	1.6	Dose adjustment may be needed in severe liver disease	[98]
		A (4)		6.70	1.3	2394	1.7		
		B (4)		8.32	2.4	1989	2.3		
		C (4)		11.05	3.1	2357	1.8		

(continued)

Table 5.3 Continued

Drug	Metabolism	Child–Pugh class (n)	PK observation CL (L/h)	AUC (ng/mL/h) (µg/mL/h)*	T½ (h)	CMax (ng/mL)	TMax (h)	Study recommendations	References
Lamotrigine	UGT1A3/4	Control (12)	1.53	66.5*	31.7	1700	1	↓ dose by 50–75% in moderate to severe cirrhosis	[99]
		B (12)	1.35	76.3	42.5	1400	1		
		C no ascites (7)	0.88	120	65	1580	1		
		C ascites (5)	0.54	197	91	1.56	2		
Lidocaine	CYP3A4	Control (10)	46		2.23			↓ dose by 50% in severe liver disease	[100]
		A (10)	47		3.15				
		C (10)	26		5.77				
Nifedipine	CYP3A4	Control (10)		↑ 2-fold	1.7	↔		Reduce dose in severe liver disease	[101]
		A/B/C (7)			7.2				
Omeprazole	CYP2C19, 3A4	Control (12)		51.8*	9.22	303		Consider dose adjustment no more than 20 mg	[102]
		A (5)		82.9					
		B (4)		96.7					
		C (4)		111.5	3.98	400			
Tacrolimus (IV)	CYP3A4	Control (6)	3.4	652	34.2	–	–	Adjust based on blood concentration	[103]
		A/B (6)	2.7	683	60.6	–	–		
Tacrolimus (Oral)		Control (8)	–	297	34.8	29.7	1.6		
		A/B (8)	–	563	66.1	48.2	1.5		
Theophylline	CYP1A2, 2E1, 3A4	Control (10)	3.3		9.3	6847	1.25	Reduce dose	[104]
		A (10)	2.7		10.6	7568	0.75		
		C (10)	1.15		30	6487	0.5		

PBC = primary biliary cirrhosis.

NB: This table is for illustrative purposes and the information presented should not be used in isolation to make clinical decisions.

Conclusion

Although knowledge of how a drug is metabolised and the effects of liver disease on these pathways will highlight drugs where caution is needed, it is often difficult to come up with definitive dosage guidelines based on these data. Routine liver function tests are generally a poor guide to the capacity of the liver to metabolise drugs, although there are specific areas where more research is needed. For instance, are the serum bilirubin level or the activity of alkaline phosphatase the best markers for dose adjustment in patients with cholestasis, or would serum bile acid be more accurate [105]? This is especially important when considering the impact of cholestasis on the kinetics and dynamics of anti-cancer drugs.

The Child–Pugh score is useful for determining short-term prognosis in patients with cirrhosis, but its usefulness for predicting drug doses is less clear. Precise determination of drug dosage in cirrhosis has to be determined on a drug-to-drug basis and requires information on changes in pharmacodynamics and plasma protein binding in addition to changes in drug elimination.

Key points

- Drug dose modification in liver disease should be considered in the following situations:
  - Drug with a narrow therapeutic range that is principally cleared by hepatic metabolism
  - Drug predominantly metabolised by CYPs 1A2, 2C19, 2D6 and 3A4
  - Prothrombin time > 130% of normal
  - Bilirubin > 100 µmol/L
  - Presence of encephalopathy
  - Presence of ascites.
- Misinterpretation of total drug concentration measurements may occur if albumin concentration is <30 g/L and the drug is > 80% bound to albumin.

References

1. Kashuba ADM, Park JJ, Persky AM, *et al.* (2006) Drug metabolism, transport and the influence of hepatic disease. In: Burton ME, Shaw LM, Schentag JJ, *et al.*, eds. *Applied Pharmacokinetics and Pharmacodynamics. Principles of*

Therapeutic Drug Monitoring, 4th edn. Baltimore: Lippincott Williams & Wilkins, pp 121–164.

2. Christensen E (2004) Prognostic models including the Child–Pugh, MELD and Mayo risk scores – where are we and where should we go? *J Hepatol* 41: 334–350.

3. Bergquist C, Lindegard J, Salmonson T (1999) Dosing recommendations in liver disease. *Clin Pharmacol Ther* 66: 201–204.

4. Ralph LD, Thomson AH, Dobbs NA, *et al.* (2003) A population model of epirubicin and application to dosage guidelines. *Cancer Chemother Pharmacol* 52: 34–40.

5. Noble S. Markham A (1995) Cyclosporine. A review of the pharmacokinetic properties, clinical efficacy and tolerability of a microemulsion-based formulation (Neoral). *Drugs* 50: 924–941.

6. MacKichan JJ (2006) Influence of protein binding and use of unbound (free) drug concentrations. In: Burton ME, Shaw LM, Schentag JJ, *et al.*, eds. *Applied Pharmacokinetics and Pharmacodynamics. Principles of Therapeutic Drug Monitoring*, 4th edn, pp 82–120. Baltimore: Lippincott Williams & Wilkins.

7. Winter ME (2004) Phenytoin. In: Winter ME. *Basic Clinical Pharmacokinetics*, 4th edn, pp 321–363. Baltimore: Lippincott Wiliams & Wilkins.

8. Blaschke TF, Meffin PJ, Melmon KL, *et al.* (1975) Influence of acute viral hepatitis on phenytoin kinetics and protein binding. *Clin Pharmacol Ther* 17: 685–691.

9. Gibaldi M, McNamara PJ (1978) Apparent volumes of distribution and drug binding to plasma proteins and tissues. *Eur J Clin Pharmacol* 13: 373–380.

10. Hasselstrom J, Eriksson S. Persson A, *et al.* (1990) The metabolism and bioavailability of morphine in patients with severe liver disease. *Br J Clin Pharmacol* 29: 289–297.

11. Nelson DR, Koymans L, Kamataki T, *et al.* (1996) P450 superfamily: update on new sequences, gene mapping, accession numbers and nomenclature. *Pharmacogenetics* 6: 1–42.

12. Shimada T, Yamazaki H, Mimura M, *et al.* (1994) Interindividual variations in human liver cytochrome P-450 enzymes involved in the oxidation of drugs, carcinogens and toxic chemicals: studies with liver microsomes of 30 Japanese and 30 Caucasians. *J Pharmacol Exp Ther* 270: 414–423.

13. Hasler JA (1999) Pharmacogenetics of cytochromes P450. *Mol Aspects Med* 20: 12–24, 25–137.

14. Tucker GT, Houston JB, Huang SM (2001) Optimizing drug development: strategies to assess drug metabolism/transporter interaction potential – towards a consensus. *Br J Clin Pharmacol* 52: 107–117.

15. Lacroix D, Sonnier M, Moncion A, *et al.* (1997) Expression of CYP3A in the human liver – evidence that the shift between CYP3A7 and CYP3A4 occurs immediately after birth. *Eur J Biochem* 247: 625–634.

16. Stevens JC, Hines RN, Gu C, *et al.* (2003) Developmental expression of the major human hepatic CYP3A enzymes. *J Pharmacol Exp Ther* 307: 573–582.

17. Pacifici GM, Kubrich M, Giuliani L, *et al.* (1993) Sulphation and glucuronidation of ritodrine in human foetal and adult tissues. *Eur J Clin Pharmacol* 44: 259–264.

18. Treluyer JM, Jacqz-Aigrain E, Alvarez F, *et al.* (1991) Expression of CYP2D6 in developing human liver. *Eur J Biochem* 202: 583–588.

19. Vieira I, Sonnier M, Cresteil T (1996) Developmental expression of CYP2E1 in the human liver. Hypermethylation control of gene expression during the neonatal period. *Eur J Biochem* 238: 476–483.

20. Alcorn J, McNamara PJ (2002) Ontogeny of hepatic and renal systemic clearance pathways in infants: part I. *Clin Pharmacokinet* 41: 959–998.

21. Sonnier M, Cresteil T (1998) Delayed ontogenesis of CYP1A2 in the human liver. *Eur J Biochem* 251: 893–898.

22. Hines RN, McCarver DG (2002) The ontogeny of human drug-metabolizing enzymes: phase 1 oxidative enzymes. *J Pharmacol Exp Ther* 300: 355–360.

23. McCarver DG, Hines RN (2002) The ontogeny of human drug-metabolizing enzymes: phase 2 conjugation enzymes and regulatory mechanisms. *J Pharmacol Exp Ther* 300: 361–366.

24. Loughnan PM, Greenwald A, Purton WW, *et al.* (1977) Pharmacokinetic observations of phenytoin disposition in the newborn and young infant. *Arch Dis Child* 52: 302–309.

25. Burtin P, Jacqz-Aigrain E, Girard P, *et al.* (1994) Population pharmacokinetics of midazolam in neonates. *Clin Pharmacol Ther* 56: 615–625.

26. Hughes J, Gill AM, Mulhearn H, *et al.* (1996) Steady-state plasma concentrations of midazolam in critically ill infants and children. *Ann Pharmacother* 30: 27–30.

27. Ellis EF, Koysooko R, Levy G (1976) Pharmacokinetics of theophylline in children with asthma. *Pediatrics* 58: 542–547.

28. Suzuki Y, Mimaki T, Cox S, *et al.* (1994) Phenytoin age–dose–concentration relationship in children. *Ther Drug Monit* 16: 145–150.

29. Summers B, Summers RS (1989) Carbamazepine clearance in paediatric epilepsy patients. Influence of body mass, dose, sex and co-medication. *Clin Pharmacokinet* 17: 208–216.

30. Blanco JG, Harrison PL, Evans WE, *et al.* (2000) Human cytochrome P450 maximal activities in pediatric versus adult liver. *Drug Metab Dispos* 28: 379–382.

31. Murry DJ, Crom WR, Reddick WE, *et al.* (1995) Liver volume as a determinant of drug clearance in children and adolescents. *Drug Metab Dispos* 23: 1110–1116.

32. Hunt A, Joel S, Dick G, *et al.* (1999) Population pharmacokinetics of oral morphine and its glucuronides in children receiving morphine as immediate-release liquid or sustained-release tablets for cancer pain. *J Pediatr* 135: 47–55.

33. Alam SN, Roberts RJ, Fischer LJ (1977) Age-related differences in salicylamide and acetaminophen conjugation in man. *J Pediatr* 90: 130–135.

34. Levy G, Khanna NN, Soda DM, *et al.* (1975) Pharmacokinetics of acetaminophen in the human neonate: formation of acetaminophen glucuronide and sulfate in relation to plasma bilirubin concentration and D-glucaric acid excretion. *Pediatrics* 55: 818–825.

35. Hoyumpa AM, Schenker S (1991) Is glucuronidation truly preserved in patients with liver disease? *Hepatol* 13: 786–795.
36. Elbekai RH, Korashy HM, El-Kadi AO (2004) The effect of liver cirrhosis on the regulation and expression of drug metabolizing enzymes. *Curr Drug Metab* 5: 157–167.
37. Villeneuve JP, Pichette V (2004) Cytochrome P450 and liver diseases. *Curr Drug Metab* 5: 273–282.
38. George J, Murray M, Byth K, *et al.* (1995) Differential alterations of cytochrome P450 proteins in livers from patients with severe chronic liver disease. *Hepatology* 21: 120–128.
39. Guengerich FP, Turvy CG (1991) Comparison of levels of several human microsomal cytochrome P-450 enzymes and epoxide hydrolase in normal and disease states using immunochemical analysis of surgical liver samples. *J Pharmacol Exp Ther* 256: 1189–1194.
40. George J, Liddle C, Murray M, *et al.* (1995) Pre-translational regulation of cytochrome P450 genes is responsible for disease-specific changes of individual P450 enzymes among patients with cirrhosis. *Biochem Pharmacol* 49: 873–881.
41. Hartleb M, Romanczyk T, Becker A, *et al.* (1992) The theophylline disposition after caffeine administration in liver cirrhosis: an index of liver function. *Ital J Gastroenterol* 24: 332–337.
42. Rodopoulos N, Wisen O, Norman A (1995) Caffeine metabolism in patients with chronic liver disease. *Scand J Clin Lab Invest* 55: 229–242.
43. Coverdale SA, Samarasinghe DA, Lin R, *et al.* (2003) Changes in antipyrine clearance and platelet count, but not conventional liver tests, correlate with fibrotic change in chronic hepatitis C: value for predicting fibrotic progression. *Am J Gastroenterol* 98: 1384–1390.
44. Sotaniemi EA, Rautio A, Backstrom M, *et al.* (1995) CYP3A4 and CYP2A6 activities marked by the metabolism of lignocaine and coumarin in patients with liver and kidney diseases and epileptic patients. *Br J Clin Pharmacol* 39: 71–76.
45. Iqbal S, Vickers C, Elias E (1990) Drug metabolism in end-stage liver disease. In vitro activities of some phase 1 and phase 2 enzymes. *J Hepatol* 11: 37–42.
46. Woodhouse KW, Mitchison HC, Mutch E, *et al.* (1985) The metabolism of 7-ethoxycoumarin in human liver microsomes and the effect of primary biliary cirrhosis: implications for studies of drug metabolism in liver disease. *Br J Clin Pharmacol* 20: 77–80.
47. Arns PA, Adedoyin A, DiBisceglie AM, *et al.* Mephenytoin disposition and serum bile acids as indices of hepatic function in chronic viral hepatitis. *Clin Pharmacol Ther* 1997; 62: 527–37.
48. Giannini E, Fasoli A, Chiarbonello B, *et al.* (2002) 13C-aminopyrine breath test to evaluate severity of disease in patients with chronic hepatitis C virus infection. *Aliment Pharmacol Ther* 16: 717–725.
49. Pique JM, Feu F, de Prada G, *et al.* (2002) Pharmacokinetics of omeprazole given by continuous intravenous infusion to patients with varying degrees of hepatic dysfunction. *Clin Pharmacokinet* 41: 999–1004.
50. Villeneuve JP, Infante-Rivard C, Ampelas M, *et al.* (1986) Prognostic value of the aminopyrine breath test in cirrhotic patients. *Hepatology* 6: 928–931.

51. Nelson E (1964) Rate of metabolism of tolbutamide in test subjects with liver disease or with impaired renal function. *Am J Med Sci* 248: 657–659.

52. Adedoyin A, Arns PA, Richards WO, *et al.* (1998) Selective effect of liver disease on the activities of specific metabolizing enzymes: investigation of cytochromes P450 2C19 and 2D6. *Clin Pharmacol Ther* 64: 8–17.

53. Lown K, Kolars J, Turgeon K, *et al.* (1992) The erythromycin breath test selectively measures P450IIIA in patients with severe liver disease. *Clin Pharmacol Ther* 51: 229–238.

54. Lee JT, Yee YG, Dorian P, *et al.* (1987) Influence of hepatic dysfunction on the pharmacokinetics of propafenone. *J Clin Pharmacol* 27: 384–389.

55. Yang LQ, Li SJ, Cao YF, *et al.* (2003) Different alterations of cytochrome P450 3A4 isoform and its gene expression in livers of patients with chronic liver diseases. *World J Gastroenterol* 9: 359–363.

56. Kleinbloesem CH, van Harten J, Wilson JP, *et al.* (1986) Nifedipine: kinetics and hemodynamic effects in patients with liver cirrhosis after intravenous and oral administration. *Clin Pharmacol Ther* 40: 21–28.

57. Chalasani N, Gorski JC, Patel NH, *et al.* (2001) Hepatic and intestinal cytochrome P450 3A activity in cirrhosis: effects of transjugular intrahepatic portosystemic shunts. *Hepatology* 34: 1103–1108.

58. MacGilchrist AJ, Birnie GG, Cook A, *et al.* (1986) Pharmacokinetics and pharmacodynamics of intravenous midazolam in patients with severe alcoholic cirrhosis. *Gut* 27: 190–195.

59. Pentikainen PJ, Valisalmi L, Himberg JJ, *et al.* (1989) Pharmacokinetics of midazolam following intravenous and oral administration in patients with chronic liver disease and in healthy subjects. *J Clin Pharmacol* 29: 272–277.

60. Somogyi A, Albrecht M, Kliems G, *et al.* (1981) Pharmacokinetics, bioavailability and ECG response of verapamil in patients with liver cirrhosis. *Br J Clin Pharmacol* 12: 51–60.

61. Cotting J, Reichen J, Kutz K, *et al.* (1990) Pharmacokinetics of isradipine in patients with chronic liver disease. *Eur J Clin Pharmacol* 38: 599–603.

62. Eichelbaum M, Mikus G, Mast V, *et al.* (1988) Pharmacokinetics and pharmacodynamics of nitrendipine in healthy subjects and patients with kidney and liver disease. *J Cardiovasc Pharmacol* 12 (Suppl 4): S6–10.

63. Farrell GC, Cooksley WG, Powell LW (1979) Drug metabolism in liver disease: activity of hepatic microsomal metabolizing enzymes. *Clin Pharmacol Ther* 26: 483–492.

64. Arrigoni A, Gindro T, Aimo G, *et al.* (1994) Monoethylglicinexylidide test: a prognostic indicator of survival in cirrhosis. *Hepatology* 20: 383–387.

65. Jost G, Wahllander A, von Mandach U, *et al.* (1987) Overnight salivary caffeine clearance: a liver function test suitable for routine use. *Hepatology* 7: 338–344.

66. Branch RA, James JA, Read AE (1976) The clearance of antipyrine and indocyanine green in normal subjects and in patients with chronic lever disease. *Clin Pharmacol Ther* 20: 81–89.

67. Mehta MU, Venkataramanan R, Burckart GJ, *et al.* (1986) Antipyrine kinetics in liver disease and liver transplantation. *Clin Pharmacol Ther* 39: 372–377.

68. Frye RF, Zgheib NK, Matzke GR, *et al.* (2006) Liver disease selectively modulates cytochrome P450-mediated metabolism. *Clin Pharmacol Ther* 80: 235–245.

69. Pichard L, Fabre I, Fabre G, *et al.* (1990) Cyclosporine A drug interactions. Screening for inducers and inhibitors of cytochrome P-450 (cyclosporine A oxidase) in primary cultures of human hepatocytes and in liver microsomes. *Drug Metab Dispos* 18: 595–606.

70. Burckart GJ, Frye RF, Kelly P, *et al.* (1998) Induction of CYP2E1 activity in liver transplant patients as measured by chlorzoxazone 6-hydroxylation. *Clin Pharmacol Ther* 63: 296–302.

71. Park JM, Lin YS, Calamia JC, *et al.* (2003) Transiently altered acetaminophen metabolism after liver transplantation. *Clin Pharmacol Ther* 73: 545–553.

72. Fleishaker JC, Ryan KK, Jansat JM, *et al.* (2001) Effect of MAO-A inhibition on the pharmacokinetics of almotriptan, an antimigraine agent in humans. *Br J Clin Pharmacol* 51: 437–441.

73. Dixon CM, Park GR, Tarbit MH (1994) Characterization of the enzyme responsible for the metabolism of sumatriptan in human liver. *Biochem Pharmacol* 47: 1253–1257.

74. Battelli mg, Musiani S, Valgimigli M, *et al.* (2001) Serum xanthine oxidase in human liver disease. *Am J Gastroenterol* 96: 1194–1199.

75. Shamma'a MH, Nasrallah SM, al-Khalidi UA (1973) Serum xanthine oxidase. An experience with 2000 patients. *Am J Dig Dis* 18: 15–22.

76. Giler S, Sperling O, Brosh S, *et al.* (1975) Serum xanthine oxidase in jaundice. *Clin Chim Acta* 63: 37–40.

77. Nuutinen HU. Activities of ethanol-metabolizing enzymes in liver diseases. *Scand J Gastroenterol* 1986; 21: 678–84.

78. Panes J, Soler X, Pares A, *et al.* (1989) Influence of liver disease on hepatic alcohol and aldehyde dehydrogenases. *Gastroenterology* 97: 708–714.

79. Pacifici GM, Viani A, Franchi M, *et al.* (1990) Conjugation pathways in liver disease. *Br J Clin Pharmacol* 30: 427–435.

80. Debinski HS, Lee CS, Danks JA, *et al.* (1995) Localization of uridine 5'-diphosphate-glucuronosyltransferase in human liver injury. *Gastroenterology* 108: 1464–1469.

81. Crotty B, Watson KJ, Desmond PV, *et al.* (1989) Hepatic extraction of morphine is impaired in cirrhosis. *Eur J Clin Pharmacol* 36: 501–506.

82. Furlan V, Demirdjian S, Bourdon O, *et al.* (1999) Glucuronidation of drugs by hepatic microsomes derived from healthy and cirrhotic human livers. *J Pharmacol Exp Ther* 289: 1169–1175.

83. Azuma T, Ito S, Suto H, *et al.* (2000) Pharmacokinetics of clarithromycin in *Helicobacter pylori* eradication therapy in patients with liver cirrhosis. *Aliment Pharmacol Ther* 14 (Suppl 1): 216–222.

84. el-Azab G, Youssef MK, Higashi Y, *et al.* (1996) Acetaminophen plasma level after oral administration in liver cirrhotic patients suffering from schistosomal infection. *Int J Clin Pharmacol Ther* 34: 299–303.

85. Chen LJ, Thaler MM, Bolt RJ, *et al.* (1978) Enzymatic sulfation of bile salts: III. enzymatic sulfation of taurolithocholate in human and guinea pig fetuses and adults. *Life Sci* 22: 1817–1820.

86. Elekima OT, Mills CO, Ahmad A, *et al.* (2000) Reduced hepatic content of dehydroepiandrosterone sulphotransferase in chronic liver diseases. *Liver* 20: 45–50.
87. Adachi Y, Horii K, Takahashi Y, *et al.* (1980) Serum glutathione *S*-transferase activity in liver diseases. *Clin Chim Acta* 106: 243–255.
88. Clemmesen JO, Tygstrup N, Ott P (1998) Hepatic plasma flow estimated according to Fick's principle in patients with hepatic encephalopathy: evaluation of indocyanine green and D-sorbitol as test substances. *Hepatology* 27: 666–673.
89. Lautt WW (1996) The 1995 Ciba-Geigy Award Lecture. Intrinsic regulation of hepatic blood flow. *Can J Physiol Pharmacol* 74: 223–233.
90. Moreno AH, Burchell AR, Rousselot LM, *et al.* (1967) Portal blood flow in cirrhosis of the liver. *J Clin Invest* 46: 436–445.
91. Wood AJ, Kornhauser DM, Wilkinson GR, *et al.* (1978) The influence of cirrhosis on steady-state blood concentrations of unbound propranolol after oral administration. *Clin Pharmacokinet* 3: 478–487.
92. Rostami-Hodjegan A, Tucker GT (2002) The effects of portal shunts on intestinal cytochrome P450 3A activity. *Hepatology* 35: 1549–1550; author reply 1550–1551.
93. Veronese L, Rautaureau J, Sadler BM, *et al.* (2000) Single-dose pharmacokinetics of amprenavir, a human immunodeficiency virus type 1 protease inhibitor, in subjects with normal or impaired hepatic function. *Antimicrob Agents Chemother* 44: 821–826.
94. Chalon SA, Desager JP, Desante KA, *et al.* (2003) Effect of hepatic impairment on the pharmacokinetics of atomoxetine and its metabolites. *Clin Pharmacol Ther* 73: 178–191.
95. Hempfling W, Grunhage F, Dilger K, *et al.* (2003) Pharmacokinetics and pharmacodynamic action of budesonide in early- and late-stage primary biliary cirrhosis. *Hepatology* 38: 196–202.
96. Slugg PH, Much DR, Smith WB, *et al.* (2000) Cirrhosis does not affect the pharmacokinetics and pharmacodynamics of clopidogrel. *J Clin Pharmacol* 40: 396–401.
97. Penenberg D, Chung M, Walmsley P, *et al.* (2000) The effects of hepatic impairment on the pharmacokinetics of doxazosin. *J Clin Pharmacol* 40: 67–73.
98. Sjovall H, Bjornsson E, Holmberg J, *et al.* (2002) Pharmacokinetic study of esomeprazole in patients with hepatic impairment. *Eur J Gastroenterol Hepatol* 14: 491–496.
99. Marcellin P, de Bony F, Garret C, *et al.* (2001) Influence of cirrhosis on lamotrigine pharmacokinetics. *Br J Clin Pharmacol* 51: 410–414.
100. Orlando R, Piccoli P, De Martin S, *et al.* (2003) Effect of the CYP3A4 inhibitor erythromycin on the pharmacokinetics of lignocaine and its pharmacologically active metabolites in subjects with normal and impaired liver function. *Br J Clin Pharmacol* 55: 86–93.
101. Ene MD, Roberts CJ (1987) Pharmacokinetics of nifedipine after oral administration in chronic liver disease. *J Clin Pharmacol* 27: 1001–1004.

102. Kumar R, Chawla YK, Garg SK, *et al.* (2003) Pharmacokinetics of omeprazole in patients with liver cirrhosis and extrahepatic portal venous obstruction. *Meth Find Exp Clin Pharmacol* 25: 625–630.

103. Bekersky I, Dressler D, Alak A, *et al.* (2001) Comparative tacrolimus pharmacokinetics: normal versus mildly hepatically impaired subjects. *J Clin Pharmacol* 41: 628–635.

104. Orlando R, Padrini R, Perazzi M, *et al.* (2006) Liver dysfunction markedly decreases the inhibition of cytochrome P450 1A2-mediated theophylline metabolism by fluvoxamine. *Clin Pharmacol Ther* 79: 489–499.

105. Delco F, Tchambaz L, Schlienger R, *et al.* (2006) Dose adjustment in patients with liver disease. *Drug Safety* 28: 529–545.

6

Undesirable side effects

Faye Croxen

Introduction

The side effect profile of many drugs is of concern in patients with liver disease. Pharmacodynamics can be altered, making effects and side effects more pronounced, e.g. heightened receptor sensitivity to anxiolytics, and the complications of liver disease, e.g. coagulopathy, may increase the risk of adverse events. This chapter discusses the types of drug that should be avoided or used with caution in patients with liver disease. A number of drugs are listed, but please note that this is not an exhaustive list and that other drugs may need to be considered (Table 6.1).

Table 6.1 Types of drugs to be used with caution/avoided in liver disease

Types of drug	Relevance in liver disease
Sedating drugs	Encephalopathy
Constipating drugs	Encephalopathy
Antiplatelets/anticoagulants	Increased risk of bleeding
Nephrotoxic drugs	Hepatorenal disease
High sodium-containing drugs	Ascites

Hepatotoxicity

Hepatotoxicity is not a particularly common form of adverse drug reaction and a patient with pre-existing liver disease does not have increased susceptibility to hepatic injury when taking drugs known to cause liver damage [1]. Therefore, drugs that are known to be hepatotoxic should not be contraindicated in this group of patients. There are a few exceptions to the general rule when greater care would be required, including hepatotoxicity with methotrexate, some chemotherapy agents and sodium valproate. If a patient with pre-existing liver disease does suffer an idiosyncratic hepatic reaction to any drug, the consequences are likely to be more severe.

It should be noted that after the administration of any drug, isolated increases in liver function tests are not proof of hepatotoxicity, and if the biochemical changes are only moderate (equivalent to an approximate increase of twice the upper limit of normal) this is unlikely to be significant [1]; however, it would be sensible to monitor liver function tests closely for further increases and to withdraw the drug if necessary. See Chapter 3 for further information on drugs that cause liver disease.

Biliary effects

If a patient has cholestasis careful consideration must be given to the use of any drug that can cause biliary problems. Several drugs are known to cause cholestatic hepatitis, including the antibiotics flucloxacillin, erythromycin and co-amoxiclav (amoxicillin/clavulanic acid). Although a patient with cholestasis is no more likely to suffer from this idiosyncratic reaction than a patient without liver impairment, it will be of greater concern if it does occur.

Biliary sludging has been documented in children receiving ceftriaxone. The formation of biliary sludge has been reported to lead to biliary obstruction, cholecystitis, choledocholithiasis and pseudolithiasis. Most cases are asymptomatic, transient, reversible, and usually only necessitate conservative management. However, greater care is required in patients with pre-existing liver disease, and it is advised that abdominal ultrasound scans are performed when ceftriaxone is initiated [2]. It would seem sensible to consider alternative antibiotic therapy in these types of patient.

Morphine has been reported to cause biliary pain by causing contraction of the sphincter of Oddi and the lower common bile duct. Other opioids may be preferred over morphine in patients with biliary pain or where biliary tract spasm is undesirable [2].

Fibrates can cause biliary lipid changes by significantly increasing the amount of cholesterol and phospholipid in the bile and reducing the amount of bile acid. A study [2] found that fibrates may be more frequently associated with the formation of gallstones compared to statins or patients not taking lipid-lowering agents. Octreotide and lanreotide have also been associated with the formation of gallstones, which is likely to be due to inhibition of gallbladder motility because of the reduced secretion of gut hormones [2].

Gastrotintestinal effects

Constipation

Drugs that are known to cause constipation should be avoided, or given with laxatives, in any patient who is encephalopathic or could become so, e.g. in acute liver failure and cirrhosis. Constipation prevents the clearance of toxic waste products in the bowel that can accumulate, cross the blood–brain barrier and cause (or worsen) encephalopathy. Examples of drugs to use with caution/avoid are:

- Opioid analgesics
- Tricyclic antidepressants
- Sedating antihistamines
- $5HT_3$ antagonists
- Calcium channel blockers
- Antispasmodics, e.g. hyoscine butylbromide
- Antimuscarinic drugs used in parkinsonism
- Aluminium-containing antacids
- Loperamide
- Anticholinergic antipsychotics (e.g. phenothiazines).

Gastrointestinal ulceration

Gastrointestinal ulceration is a considerable risk in patients with portal hypertension, varices, deranged clotting (high INR/PT) or low platelets. The integrity of the gastrointestinal mucosa can be affected by excessive alcohol consumption [3] and may increase the risk of gastrointestinal ulceration. Drugs with this side effect profile should, if possible, be avoided in these types of patient. Examples of drugs to use with caution/ avoid are:

- Non-steroidal anti-inflammatories (NSAIDs)
- Aspirin
- Corticosteroids
- Bisphosphonates.

Neurological effects

Sedation

Drugs that affect the central nervous system (CNS) should be used with caution or avoided in patients at risk of developing encephalopathy. Tissue responsiveness to the pharmacological action of some drugs may be modified, as evidenced by the increased susceptibility of the brain, in patients with cirrhosis, to the action of many psychoactive drugs [4]. If the metabolic capacity of the liver is impaired, e.g. in acute liver failure or cirrhosis, the patient may be, or become, encephalopathic. In encephalopathy the brain is more sensitive to the sedating effects of any drug due to altered blood–brain permeability, cerebral blood flow and receptor sensitivity. In particular, the CNS side effects of certain drugs, such as sedation and confusion, can increase the risk or worsen the grade of encephalopathy by compounding the CNS depressant effects [5]. The potential for drug accumulation in these types of patient, as a result of reduced metabolism or excretion, further increases the risk of side effects occurring. Examples of sedating drugs to use with caution/ avoid are:

- Opioid analgesics
- Tricyclic antidepressants
- Sedating antihistamines
- Benzodiazepines and other hypnotics
- Barbiturates
- Antipsychotics (e.g. phenothiazines).

Seizures

Tramadol, phenothiazine antipsychotics and the majority of anti-depressants, as well as a number of other drugs, can lower the seizure threshold and are associated with an increased risk of convulsions [6]. Again, these drugs may accumulate in patients with liver impairment such as cirrhosis or acute liver failure, and care must be taken if choosing to use them. This is especially important in alcoholics, who have an increased risk of seizures from acute alcohol withdrawal [7]. Examples of drugs that can lower the seizure threshold and should be used with caution/avoided are:

- Tramadol
- Pethidine
- Antidepressants

- Sedating antihistamines
- Antipsychotics (e.g. phenothiazines).

Endocrine/metabolic effects

Drugs that can disturb fluid–electrolyte balance must be used with caution in patients with certain types of liver impairment. Diuretics, for example, are often required to treat ascites but can cause hyponatraemia, hypo- or hyperkalaemia. A disturbance in electrolyte balance can lead to encephalopathy in susceptible patients such as cirrhotics or those with acute liver failure. Dehydration induced by diuretics is a common precipitant of hepatic encephalopathy. The mechanism is not fully understood, but could possibly be due to the reduced metabolism of hepatic toxins because of hepatic hypoxia [5].

The clearance of lactate may be reduced in liver impairment, leading to the possibility of accumulation and increased potential for lactic acidosis. Concurrent renal impairment with liver impairment could further increase the risk with drugs known to cause lactic acidosis, e.g. metformin and nucleoside reverse transcriptase inhibitors [2].

Some drugs may worsen ascites, for example those with a high sodium content. Examples of drugs to use with caution/avoid are:

- Diuretics
- Sodium-containing medications and intravenous solutions
- Soluble tablets containing high levels of sodium
- Metformin
- Nucleoside reverse transcriptase inhibitors.

Haematological effects

Bleeding

Coagulopathy is a common complication of liver disease. Synthesis of vitamin K and clotting factors is impaired in patients with cirrhosis and acute liver failure. Cirrhosis can also cause a reduced platelet synthesis of thromboxane-2, and a platelet adhesion defect is sometimes seen [8]. Cholestatic patients may have deranged clotting due to vitamin K malabsorption.

Several studies have reported bleeding disorders associated with the use of selective serotonin reuptake inhibitors (SSRIs). This is considered to be the result of a decrease in the uptake of serotonin into platelets, leading to a reduced ability to form clots and a subsequent increase in the risk of bleeding. Published clinical evidence looking at the risk of gastrointestinal bleeding with SSRIs is limited to observational studies, but available evidence shows that concurrent use of NSAIDs or aspirin with SSRIs increases the risk of upper gastrointestinal bleeding [9].

Any drug that can increase the risk of bleeding must be used with caution or avoided in patients with liver impairment associated with deranged clotting, portal hypertension, varices or low platelets. Examples of such drugs are:

- NSAIDs
- Aspirin
- Clopidogrel
- Dipyridamole
- Warfarin
- Heparin
- SSRIs
- Corticosteroids
- Drugs that cause thrombocytopenia.

Dermatological effects

Patients with cholestatic conditions such as gallstones, primary sclerosing cholangitis or Alagille's syndrome often suffer from pruritus that can be extremely debilitating. In such patients it would seem sensible to avoid medication that could exacerbate this symptom. Administration of opiates via the intrathecal and epidural routes lead to a high incidence of pruritus (up to 80% with epidural morphine) [2].

Renal effects

Patients with liver impairment, such as cirrhosis with portal hypertension (particularly alcoholic cirrhosis/hepatitis) or acute liver failure, are more susceptible to renal impairment than those without liver impairment. Care should be taken with any drug that is potentially nephrotoxic or could contribute to renal dysfunction in these types of patients.

Portal hypertension in cirrhotic patients leads to arterial vasodilation in the splanchnic circulation, owing to an increased production of nitric oxide and other vasodilatory substances. This results in a low peripheral vascular resistance and a hyperdynamic circulation, with the development of arterial hypotension. In order to compensate for this the renin–angiotensin and sympathetic nervous systems are activated, leading to vasoconstriction in extra-splanchnic vascular areas such as the kidneys. This extreme renal vasoconstriction results in very low renal perfusion and glomerular filtration rate (GFR), and a reduced ability to excrete sodium and free water. This condition is known as hepatorenal syndrome and is a frequent complication of advanced cirrhosis [10, 11].

It is difficult to obtain an accurate measure of renal function in patients with cirrhosis. A number of studies have shown that they tend to have low serum creatinine levels. This has been explained by a reduced muscle mass in cirrhotic patients and a reduced conversion of creatine to creatinine [10]. The calculation of creatinine clearance using the Cockcroft and Gault formula is also inaccurate in predicting GFR in these patients because it uses the serum creatinine level (which may be falsely low) and body weight in the calculation, which is likely to be inflated due to the presence of ascites [12]. The measured creatinine clearance, based on urinary excretion of creatinine, should theoretically be more accurate, even in patients with reduced muscle mass or impaired creatinine synthesis. However, it has been shown that this also overestimates the GFR because of an increased fractional tubular secretion of creatinine in cirrhotic patients, particularly those with reduced GFR [10].

Because GFR is usually decreased in patients with cirrhosis and assessments-based creatinine clearance can greatly overestimate renal drug clearance, drugs with considerable renal elimination and those with a narrow therapeutic range should be prescribed with caution [10].

The administration of NSAIDs can cause a significant decrease in renal function. They reduce the formation of prostaglandins, and in doing so can decrease GFR in susceptible patients. Those with cirrhosis and ascites are at the greatest risk of developing renal impairment with NSAIDs, as they are highly reliant on prostaglandins for maintenance of their renal blood flow and renal function compared to other patients [13, 14]. It may also be prudent to avoid cyclo-oxygenase (COX)-2 inhibitors in these susceptible patients because, although there are no clinical trials in patients with liver disease, they have been shown to reduce renal perfusion in salt-depleted healthy subjects [10].

Examples of drugs to use with caution/avoid are:

- NSAIDs
- COX-2 inhibitors
- Aminoglycosides

- Diuretics
- ACE inhibitors
- Iodine-containing contrast agents.

Herbal/recreational drugs

Herbal medicines are becoming more and more popular, and indeed some herbal products may be considered to benefit people with liver disease, e.g. *Silybum marianum* (milk thistle), *Picrorhiza kurroa*, *Phyllanthus*, etc. Herbal hepatotoxicity is increasingly being recognised, for example, with kava kava, black cohosh, and many traditional Chinese remedies. The range of liver injury includes minor transaminase elevations, acute and chronic hepatitis, steatosis, cholestasis, zonal or diffuse hepatic necrosis, veno-occlusive disease and acute liver failure. In addition to the potential for hepatotoxicity, herb–drug interactions may affect the safety and efficacy of concurrent medical therapy [15].

Because of an incomplete understanding of their modes of action, lack of standardisation in their manufacture and limited awareness of potential adverse effects, great care must be taken in using herbal medicines in patients with liver disease, and often the safest option is simply to avoid them because of the lack of information. This statement can also be applied to recreational drugs.

References

1. Farrell GC (ed) (1994) *Drug-induced Liver Disease*. London: Churchill Livingstone.
2. Hutchinson TA, Shahan DR, Anderson ML (eds) Drugdex System internet version. Micromedex Inc. Colorado: Greenwood Village. (Accessed May 2007.)
3. Chou S (1994) An examination of the alcohol consumption and peptic ulcer association – results of a national survey. *Alcohol Clin Exp Res* 18: 149–153.
4. Westphal JF, Brogard JM (1997) Drug administration in chronic liver disease. *Drug Safety* 17: 47–73.
5. Riordan S, Williams R (1997) Treatment of hepatic encephalopathy. *N Engl J Med* 337: 473–479.
6. *British National Formulary*, 52nd edn. (2006) London: BMJ Publishing and RPS Publishing.
7. Brathen G, Ben-Menachem E, Brodtkorb E *et al.* (2005) EFNS guideline on the diagnosis and management of alcohol-related seizures: report of an EFNS task force. *Eur J Neurol* 12: 575–581.
8. Laffi G, Cominelli F (1988) Altered platelet function in cirrhosis of the liver: Impairment of inositol lipid and arachidonic acid metabolism in response to agonists. *Hepatology* 8: 1620–1626.

9. Paton C, Ferrier N (2005) SSRIs and gastrointestinal bleeding. *Br Med J* 331: 529–530.

10. Delco F, Tchambaz L, Schlienger R, Drewe J, Krahenbuhl S (2005) Dose adjustments in patients with liver disease. *Drug Safety* 28: 529–545.

11. Arroyo V, Terra C, Gines P (2007) Advances in the pathogenesis and treatment of type-1 and type-2 hepatorenal syndrome. *J Hepatol* 46: 935–946.

12. Morgan J, Mclean A (1995) Clinical pharmacokinetic and pharmacodynamic considerations in patients with liver disease. *Clin Pharmacokinet* 29: 370–391.

13. Gentilini P, Laffi G (1989) Renal functional impairment and sodium retention in liver cirrhosis. *Digestion* 43: 1–32.

14. Laffi G (1997) Arachidonic acid derivatives and renal function in liver cirrhosis. *Semin Nephrol* 17: 530–548.

15. Stedman C (2002) Herbal hepatotoxicity. *Semin Liver Dis* 22: 195–206.

Part Three

Putting the theory into practice

7

Applying the principles – introduction

Janet Tweed

Can you use paracetamol in a patient with liver disease?

If you have answered 'yes' or 'no' to this question, think again! Many people would answer no, perhaps because of the worries about paracetamol hepatotoxicity. The answer, however, is most likely to be yes, but in actual fact you cannot answer it without knowing more about the patient. The question is too vague. Chapters 1 to 6 explain why this is the case and give you the background information to enable you to adequately consider drug choice in patients with liver dysfunction.

Why is the question too vague?

Apart from the usual questions (for example, is paracetamol an appropriate analgesic for the type of pain?), we do not know enough about the breadth and severity of the liver disease. This is key information when deciding whether a particular drug can be used, and therefore it is very difficult to generalise and answer a non-patient-specific enquiry. Further information on the assessment of liver function and how this relates to drug handling can be found in Chapter 4.

Once you appreciate the complexity of the above question and the need for further information, you should find this final part of the book useful in putting all the theory you have learnt into practice.

Part 3 Outline

Chapter 7

- How will this section help you?
- Introduction to the five patient cases

- Introduction to the treatment choice scenarios
- How should you use this section?
- Applying the principles to your patient: what information do you need, and where can you find it?
  - Type, extent and severity of liver disease
  - Non-liver-related patient-specific factors
  - Drug-related information
    - Short-cuts to finding relevant information
    - Clinical studies
    - First principles
      - Pharmacokinetics and pharmacodynamics
      - Adverse effects
      - Interactions.

Chapter 8
- The *aide mémoire*

Chapter 9
- Scenario 1 – Choice of analgesia

Chapter 10
- Scenario 2 – Choice of antiemetic

Chapter 11
- Scenario 3 – Choice of anti-hyperlipidaemic agent

Chapter 12
- Scenario 4 – Choice of hormone replacement therapy (HRT)

Chapter 13
- Scenario 5 – Choice of contraceptive

Appendix 1
- Detailed description of the five patient cases

Appendix 2
- Blank *aide mémoire* form.

How will this section help you?

This third and final part of the book uses patient-specific cases to illustrate why different types of liver disease or dysfunction affect drug handling in different ways. It brings together the information contained in the previous chapters to clearly demonstrate the relevance of all of the following when choosing a drug therapy or contemplating the appropriateness of an existing drug therapy in a patient with liver dysfunction (Figure 7.1):

1. Type, extent and severity of liver disease
2. Pharmacokinetics and pharmacodynamics of the drug

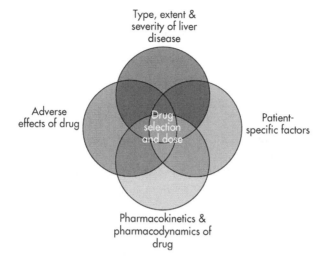

Figure 7.1 Factors to consider when deciding on optimum drug treatment for a patient with liver dysfunction.

3. Adverse reactions of the drug
4. Patient-specific factors.

The following list, which is not exhaustive, gives some examples of non-liver-related, patient-specific considerations:

- Age of patient
- Past medical history
- Comorbidities
- Drug history
- Concomitant medications
- Allergies
- Severity of the condition to be treated
- Preferred route of drug administration
- Renal function.

The cases have kept these patient-specific details to a minimum, in order to focus on the hepatic aspects of each scenario. The scenarios should therefore not be used to provide definitive answers to the questions asked, as there will undoubtedly be many other pertinent factors to take into account in your patient. Instead, they should be used to learn about the principles involved when choosing drug therapy for patients with different types of liver dysfunction.

There is no right or wrong order when working through the four considerations listed above. However, it is advisable to obtain all patient-related information first, before moving on to the characteristics of potential drug treatments.

In some circumstances it may be more appropriate to consider the non-liver-related patient-specific factors first. For example, when choosing an analgesic for a patient with liver dysfunction and a past history of gastric ulcer, you may wish to exclude non-steroidal anti-inflammatory drugs (NSAIDs) from your treatment options from the start. In other situations, particularly when you become more familiar with drug choices in patients with hepatic dysfunction, it may be easier to initially disregard drugs from a liver disease perspective. For example, when choosing drugs in decompensated cirrhotic patients it is preferable to avoid sedating drugs.

Introduction to the five patient cases

In order to demonstrate the drug-handling issues that are relevant in different types of liver disease, five patients are discussed. Each patient has a specific diagnosis, which serves as an example of a specific type of liver dysfunction. Even if your patient does not have the same diagnosis as one of these examples, their pattern of liver dysfunction, and hence their drug handling, is likely to be similar to one of the five. Full details of each case can be found in Appendix 1.

The five patients are as follows:

Patient	Diagnosis	Type/pattern of liver dysfunction
Patient 1	Non-alcoholic steatohepatitis	Mild hepatitis without cirrhosis
Patient 2	Primary sclerosing cholangitis	Cholestasis
Patient 3	Cryptogenic cirrhosis	Compensated cirrhosis
Patient 4	Alcoholic liver disease	Decompensated cirrhosis
Patient 5	Paracetamol overdose	Acute liver failure

Introduction to the treatment choice scenarios

All the scenarios describe why each of the five patients has different issues that should be taken into account when considering drug choice, thus demonstrating the importance of knowing as much as you can about the patient's liver disease. The scenarios are not all-encompassing and do not include all potential drug treatments. Drugs are included in the options purely to demonstrate some of the principles involved.

Each case scenario begins with a summary, outlining drug-related information pertinent to the use of the drug(s) in patients with liver dysfunction. After the summary there is a more detailed review of the available data, describing the following information:

Section title	Comments/considerations	Sources of information unless otherwise specified (full citations at end of chapter)
Pharmacokinetics	Considers: Absorption Distribution Metabolism Elimination A summary of relevant facts which may be incomplete, depending on the data available	References 1–6 and Summaries of Product Characteristics (SPC)
Pharmacodynamics	Changes in receptor sensitivity. Changes in pharmacological effect	References 1–5 and SPC
Some relevant adverse effects	Considers: Hepatotoxicity Biliary effects Gastrointestinal effects Neurological effects Endocrine/metabolic effects Haematological effects Dermatological effects Renal effects	References 1, 3–5, 7–10 and SPC (Drug Analysis Print data – adverse drug reactions reported to the MHRA* – have been excluded as they are not generally needed)
Some relevant drug reactions	List not exhaustive Includes only those drug interactions that potentially affect the handling of the drug by the liver	References 1, 5, 6, and SPC
Clinical studies	Includes published studies and case reports describing the use of the drug(s) in patients with various types of liver disease Includes paediatric studies where available	Reference 5 and Medline/Embase searches

*Medicines and Healthcare Products Regulatory Agency.

Each scenario ends with the application of this drug-related information to the five patient cases, and a recommendation as to which treatment(s) may be the preferred option(s) and/or which to avoid.

How should you use this section?

You can use this part of the book in two ways:

1.   As a learning tool. Read through all the cases to expand your knowledge and awareness of pertinent issues.
2.   To help you apply the principles to a patient of your own.

For the latter:

• Obtain as much information as possible about your patient's liver function, and use this to assess the type, extent and severity of liver disease or dysfunction. You may find the *aide mémoire* in the Appendix helpful to remind you of the relevant data.
• Using this information, find the patient case that most closely resembles your patient's pattern of liver dysfunction. Use the possible alternative diagnoses section at the end of each case to help you.
• Read all the scenarios for the matching patient case, in order to gain a practical understanding of the principles that are relevant in that type of patient.
• Obtain all other pertinent patient-specific factors that may influence your choice of treatment. Do not forget about other pathologies they may have.
• Use the section below (Applying the principles to your patient: what information do you need to obtain and where can you find it?) to help you obtain other applicable information, including the characteristics of the drugs you are considering using.
• Apply the principles you have learnt from previous chapters and from the case scenarios to your patient when reviewing their drug treatment, ensuring that you consider all the information you have obtained.

Applying the principles to your patient: what information do you need to obtain and where can you find it?

You may find it useful to complete the *aide mémoire* located in Appendix 2 before you start researching your question.

   Many reference sources are quoted in this section. The full citations are given at the end of this introduction.

Type, extent and severity of liver disease

Some of the information (discussed previously in Chapter 4) needed to assess liver function can be found in the patient's medical notes (e.g. laboratory results). However, it is generally useful to speak to an appropriate clinician to obtain more specific information relating to results of scans, specialist tests and investigations, etc. The opinion of a specialist regarding the extent, severity and possible causes of the liver dysfunction is often invaluable.

Non-liver-related patient-specific factors

These are generally identified by examining the patient's medical notes, and through discussion with the patient and/or their doctor.

Drug-related information

Short-cuts to finding relevant information

Sometimes the British National Formulary (BNF) [1] or the Summary of Product Characteristics (SPC) endorses the use of a drug in patients with liver disease. This is often sufficient and no further research is required. However, ensure that you also check the adverse effects of the drug, as these may preclude its use in some patients, even if there are no explicit contraindications or precautions regarding liver disease in the SPC.

If the BNF and SPC *do* contraindicate or caution against the use of the drug in liver disease, then further investigation and research is generally needed. This is because the recommendation may be based on a lack of or inconclusive data, rather than adverse data. In these situations, application of knowledge from first principles is often appropriate, and a risk–benefit assessment for your specific patient should be considered. Use of drugs outside their product licence may be considered appropriate in some situations.

Clinical studies

Information regarding the pharmacokinetic/dynamic profile of a drug and its potential side effects allows you to consider, *from first principles*, whether that drug is appropriate to use in a specific patient with liver disease, or whether it is best avoided. However, it is sometimes unnecessary to work solely from first principles: other researchers may have already carried out and published some of this work for you. It is therefore useful to perform a literature search in order to identify any relevant studies that examine use of the drug in question in patients with similar types of liver disease to that of your patient.

First principles

Pharmacokinetics and pharmacodynamics
Being familiar with the pharmacokinetic and pharmacodynamic profile of a drug enables you to assess how the handling of that drug may be affected in a patient with impaired hepatic function (see Chapter 5 for more detail).

Basic pharmacokinetic/dynamic information can be found in a number of common sources such as the BNF, the SPC for the drug (or equivalent data if outside the UK), *Martindale: The Complete Drug Reference* and *AHFS Drug Information* [1,3,4]. There are other books, such as *Therapeutic Drugs,* edited by C. Dollery, which may give more detailed information [2]. Other useful sources include online pharmacy and medical databases, bibliographic databases to identify relevant published material, and pharmaceutical manufacturers.

Adverse effects
Relevant adverse effects are discussed in Chapter 6. It is important to determine whether the drug you are considering can cause any of these effects, and if so, the severity and the likelihood of those effect(s) occurring. This information will influence the risk–benefit assessment of the use of the medication in your patient. In addition, if you choose to use a drug that has potential associated risks, you will need to know which adverse effects to look out for, to ensure safe treatment. For example, which side effects suggest accumulation, which signs/symptoms/test results suggest hepatotoxicity?

Adverse drug reaction (ADR) data can be found in a number of sources. Useful resources to start your search include the BNF, SPC, *Martindale* and *AHFS Drug Information* [1,3,4].

In many instances the above sources will give you sufficient data. However, sometimes you may need more detailed information relating to risk factors, incidence, severity, etc. This may be useful when choosing between two drugs which have similar adverse effects profiles, or when trying to identify whether a patient's liver disease is due to an existing drug treatment. The UK Medicines Information Service (www.ukmi.nhs.uk) has a recommended essential resources list containing textbooks and online sources. Included in this list are specific adverse drug reaction resources, and these may add further detail to the information you have collected so far. There are a number of hepatotoxicity books on the market that give specific detail on these types of reaction. Such books are not generally available to most pharmacy departments, although some specialist services may keep them. Other sources of ADR information include online pharmacy and medical databases, bibliographic databases to identify relevant published reports, and pharmaceutical manufacturers. It is rarely necessary to access data reported to regulatory authorities, e.g. *Drug Analysis Prints* in the UK (suspected adverse drug reactions reported to the MHRA), unless you are specifically trying to identify whether a drug could have caused a specific hepatotoxic reaction in a patient.

Interactions

Drug interactions are not specifically listed as one of the four factors that should be considered when optimising drug treatment in patients with liver dysfunction. However, it is useful to be aware of certain types of drug interaction that may be relevant. Of particular importance are those relating to enzyme induction or inhibition. Some patients with liver disease may already have a reduced capacity to metabolise drugs, potentially leading to accumulation. If these patients are also taking two interacting drugs, the interaction being due to enzyme inhibition or induction, then the effect the liver dysfunction will have on the removal of a drug from the body will be less predictable. Similarly, other pharmacokinetic interactions may complicate the picture in patients with liver disease, for example interactions affecting absorption in patients with cholestasis or ascites. The significance of these interactions is always increased unpredictability!

Pharmacodynamic 'interactions' may also be relevant to patients with liver disease. These generally occur when two drugs having the same pharmacological effect are given together and cause additive or synergistic effects. It is often the additive *adverse* effects that need to be taken into consideration in patients with liver disease, for example sedation or constipation in patients predisposed to encephalopathy.

Again, the BNF and SPC are useful in identifying pharmacokinetic drug interactions [1]. *Stockley's Drug Interactions* [6] may give more detail on the mechanism, if required. Pharmacodynamic drug interactions do not always come under the strict definition of drug interactions; however, checking for additive pharmacological and adverse effects in the resources listed under 'Adverse effects' above should identify these.

References

1.   Mehta DK (ed) (2007) *British National Formulary*. No. 53. London: British Medical Association and the Royal Pharmaceutical Society of Great Britain.

2. Dollery C (ed) (1999), *Therapeutic Drugs,* 2nd edn. London: Churchill Livingstone.
3. Sweetman S (ed) (2006) *Martindale: The Complete Drug Reference,* 35th edn. London: Pharmaceutical Press.
4. McEvoy GK (ed) (2007) *AHFS Drug Information 2007.* Bethesda, MA: American Society of Health-System Pharmacists.
5. Hutchison TA, Shahan DR, Anderson ML (eds) *Drugdex System* Internet version Micromedex Inc. Colorado: Greenwood Village.
6. Baxter I (ed) (2005) *Stockley's Drug Interactions,* 7th edn. London: Pharmaceutical Press.
7. Aronson JK (ed) (2006) *Meyler's Side Effects of Drugs: The International Encyclopedia of Adverse Drug Reactions and Interactions,* 15th edn. Amsterdam: Elsevier.
8. Zimmerman HJ (ed) (1999) *Hepatotoxicity – the Adverse Effects of Drugs and Other Chemicals on the Liver,* 2nd edn. Baltimore: Lippincott Williams & Wilkins.
9. Farrell GC (ed) (1994) *Drug-induced Liver Disease.* London: Churchill Livingstone.
10. Stricker BHCH (1992) *Drug-induced Hepatic Injury,* 2nd edn. Amsterdam: Elsevier.

8

The *aide mémoire*

Penny North-Lewis

There is little information available on drug handling in patients with liver dysfunction, so we often have to go back to first principles. What we are looking for are patient-specific factors that might affect the pharmacokinetics of a drug and drug-specific factors that may increase the risk of using the drug in our patient. This *aide mémoire* has been designed to help you consider those factors. It should only be required after standard sources such as the *British National Formulary* [1] or the *Summary of Product Characteristics* have cautioned against the use of the drug in liver disease, although you should be aware of the side effect profile of a drug, which may preclude its use in some liver patients, even if it is not specifically contraindicated, e.g. NSAIDs (see Chapter 9).

To use the *aide mémoire* you should complete the first page, gathering information about your patient, and from this determine what you need to consider in more detail with regard to the drug. There is a blank copy in Appendix 2.

Step 1: Gathering patient information

See Chapter 4 for more detailed information about the tests, signs and symptoms of liver disease.

Diagnosis

This is helpful because it gives you clues as to what sort of liver picture you should expect to see in your patient. For example, if they have auto-immune hepatitis they will have a hepatic picture of liver dysfunction, which could range from mild fibrosis with fairly normal liver function to cirrhosis which may be decompensated – you can look for signs and symptoms to help you decide how advanced their liver disease is.

Relevant biochemical tests

It is helpful to have results for all of the tests listed if they are available. It is also beneficial to see what the trend is and to indicate whether it is static or changing (improving or worsening). Perhaps use two up arrows if the biochemical result is increasing rapidly: for example, in someone with acute liver failure ALT may be doubling each day, whereas for a well-compensated patient with cirrhosis it may not have changed significantly for many months. A split bilirubin may not be available, but is useful if your patient is cholestatic as it indicates whether the bilirubin is high because of increased production or reduced clearance. Increased production is unlikely to have an impact on drug handling, although it may cause displacement from protein-binding sites: reduced clearance may affect drugs that are cleared via the biliary system. Many of these tests can be altered in conditions unrelated to liver disease, and it is important to rule these out, e.g. low albumin from malnutrition, nephropathy or enteropathy; raised INR due to warfarin therapy; raised ALP in bone disease.

Signs of liver disease and useful test results likely to have an impact on drug handling

It is probably unnecessary to gather information on all the signs and symptoms a patient may have, although they help give a better overall picture of the severity of their liver disease. The signs listed could, however, have a direct impact on drug handling, and you should find out whether your patient has them.

- Gynaecomastia, unless related to spironolactone use, indicates that the liver's metabolising capacity is reduced as it is unable to metabolise oestrogens.
- Ascites affects the volume of distribution of water-soluble drugs and may impair oral absorption of drugs, as the bowel may be oedematous.
- Varices indicate that portal vein blood flow has been diverted away from the liver secondary to portal hypertension. This would have a significant impact on first-pass metabolism, increasing the bioavailability of oral drugs that are usually extensively cleared on first pass through the liver, i.e. those with a high extraction ratio (>0.7).
- Failure to thrive/weight loss indicates a combination of problems in relation to high catabolism and poor absorption of fats due to cholestasis. Where the latter is implicated this may affect oral absorption of highly lipid-soluble drugs, requiring larger doses, alternative routes or alternative drugs to be considered.

- Encephalopathy is a sign of advanced liver disease, either acute or chronic. It usually means that there is altered mechanics across the blood–brain barrier, probably increasing permeability and cerebral blood flow. As a result, patients are more susceptible to CNS side effects of drugs. There is also evidence that the pharmacodynamics, i.e. the receptor sensitivity, of drugs may be altered.
- Pale stools indicate partial or complete (if the stools are white) blockage of the bile ducts, such that reduced or no bile is excreted. This will affect the absorption of highly lipophilic drugs, e.g. fat-soluble vitamins, as no bile salts will be secreted into the duodenum to solubilise fats. It will also mean that drugs that are cleared exclusively by the biliary system will have significantly reduced clearance.
- Jaundice indicates that the total serum bilirubin is raised: above 50 µmol/L in adults or 80 µmol/L in neonates.

Tests

Your patient may have only had some of the following tests performed. Many of them are different ways of extracting the same information.

- Biopsy results, where available, are invaluable. They may have been taken to help diagnose a disease or to give an indication of its progression. Either way, they enable you to differentiate between a mild hepatitis with an ALT of 100 and cirrhosis with a similar transaminase level. This is very helpful in determining whether or not hepatocyte function is likely to be impaired. It may also demonstrate poor biliary canaliculi or portal tracts which may result in defective bile or blood flow.
- ERCP/HIDA results will provide information regarding bile flow and any mechanical problems identified. They may be useful for highlighting the degree of cholestasis.
- Ultrasound, particularly Doppler ultrasound, provides an indication of blood flow through the liver and whether that flow is reversed. This is another way of identifying whether first-pass metabolism is likely to be affected by collateral blood flow bypassing the liver. The scan may also show whether the liver is large and inflamed (hepatitis) or small and knobbly (cirrhosis).
- Endoscopy shows whether or not oesophageal or gastric varices are present, and hence whether collateral vessels have formed, affecting blood flow through the liver.
- The encephalopathy score gives an indication of how severe the liver impairment is. A score of 1 shows early signs of liver decompensation; a score of 4 implies end-stage liver failure with very little function remaining.

• MELD/PELD/Child–Pugh scores are not designed to provide information on likely drug handling in a patient, but they are often used as surrogate markers in clinical trials. If available, they may give an indication of how far advanced the liver disease is overall.

By gathering the information above you should be able to decide which aspects of the patient's liver disease are of concern with regard to drug handling.

Examples

Patient 1 Patient Information
Name/DoB/unit number: Anna Bell, 27 years old
Diagnosis (type/cause) (if known): Unknown ?drug induced
Relevant biochemical tests:

Test	Result – recent changes ↑ ↓ ↔	Normal range
ALT/AST	35↔	<40 IU/L
Bilirubin	120 ↑	5–21 µmol/L
Split bilirubin*	101 conjugated ↑	<4 µmol/L
Alk phos	780 ↑	70–300 IU/L
GGT	N/A	<40 IU/L
Albumin	42 ↔	34–48 g/L
INR/PT	1.1 ↔	0.9–1.2
Creatinine/creatinine clearance/GFR**	79 ↔	70–100 µmol/L

Caution: Check for non-liver causes of abnormal results, e.g. warfarin, bone disease.
* May be useful in determining reason for hyperbilirubinaemia – not a routine test.
** Caution with interpreting in cirrhotic patients.

Signs of liver disease and useful test results likely to have an impact on drug handling

Sign	Present?	Tests	Result
Gynaecomastia		Biopsy	Cholestasis
Ascites		ERCP/HIDA	No excretion
Varices		Ultrasound scan – Doppler	Dilated bile ducts
Failure to thrive/ wt loss	Small	Endoscopy	N/A
Pale stools	✓	MELD/PELD/ Child–Pugh	N/A
Encephalopathy		Encephalopathy score/grade	None

Using all the information available, including the signs and test results, tick which apply with severity or grade if known

Effect on kinetics/dynamics		Risk factors for side effects	
Ascites (A/D)		Varices	
Cholestasis (A/E)	✓	Coagulopathy or low platelets	
Low albumin (D)		Encephalopathy	
Portal hypertension (M)		Pruritus	✓
Acute liver failure (M)		Alcoholism	
Cirrhosis – compensated (M)		Ascites	
Cirrhosis – decompensated (M)		Renal impairment/hepatorenal	
Encephalopathy (P)		Cirrhosis	

A = absorption; D = distribution; M = metabolism; E = elimination; P = pharmacodynamics.

Patient 1 has been gradually becoming more cholestatic over the last few weeks. Her results suggest that because of the cholestasis the absorption of lipid-soluble drugs and the elimination of biliary cleared drugs may be affected. She has pruritus associated with the cholestasis, so drugs that cause itching are best avoided.

Patient 2 Patient Information
Name/DoB/unit number: Colin Day, 43 years old
Diagnosis (type/cause) (if known): Cryptogenic cirrhosis
Relevant biochemical tests:

Test	Result – recent changes ↑ ↓ ↔	Normal range
ALT/AST	64 ↔	<60 IU/L
Bilirubin	35 ↔	5–21 µmol/L
Split bilirubin*	N/A	
Alk phos	595 ↔	70–300 IU/L
GGT	N/A	<40 IU/L
Albumin	34 ↓ (but slowly)	34–48 g/L
INR/PT	1.3 ↔	0.9–1.2
Creatinine/creatinine clearance/GFR**	98 ↔	80–115 µmol/L

Caution: Check for non-liver causes of abnormal results, e.g. warfarin, bone disease.
* May be useful in determining reason for hyperbilirubinaemia – not a routine test.
** Caution with interpreting in cirrhotic patients.

Signs of liver disease and useful test results likely to have an impact on drug handling

Sign	Present?	Tests	Result
Gynaecomastia		Biopsy	Cirrhosis
Ascites		ERCP/HIDA	N/A
Varices	✓	Ultrasound scan – Doppler	Reduced flow in PV. Nodular liver
Failure to thrive/ wt loss	✓	Endoscopy	Grade 1 varices
Pale stools		MELD/PELD/ Child–Pugh	N/A
Encephalopathy		Encephalopathy score/grade	None

Using all the information available, including the signs and test results, tick which apply with severity or grade if known

Effect on kinetics/dynamics		Risk factors for side effects	
Ascites (A/D)		Varices	✓
Cholestasis (A/E)		Coagulopathy or low platelets	?✓
Low albumin (D)	✓	Encephalopathy	?✓
Portal hypertension (M)	✓	Pruritus	
Acute liver failure (M)		Alcoholism	
Cirrhosis – compensated (M)	✓	Ascites	
Cirrhosis – decompensated (M)		Renal impairment/hepatorenal	?✓
Encephalopathy (P)		Cirrhosis	✓

A = absorption; D = distribution; M = metabolism; E = elimination; P = pharmacodynamics.

Patient 2 has raised LFTs but all less than twice the upper limit of normal. His varices are managed with regular courses of sclerotherapy. The ultrasound scan shows a small nodular liver with reduced blood flow in the portal vein on Doppler. He has a slightly low albumin (highly protein-bound drugs may need a dosage adjustment) and portal hypertension (first-pass metabolism may be reduced). His biopsy indicates cirrhosis, but his liver's synthetic function is good, with a near normal INR, albumin and bilirubin, and he has no encephalopathy; he has compensated cirrhosis and consequently should have fairly normal hepatocyte function. Because of his varices drugs that cause GI irritation or affect coagulation or platelet function should be used with caution or avoided. Although this patient does not have signs of encephalopathy it is important to remember that someone with compensated liver cirrhosis can decompensate at any time and that drug side effects may be responsible, and so drugs which are sedating or constipating should only be used cautiously and with regular review to ensure they are discontinued if the patient deteriorates. Finally, renally toxic drugs should be avoided if possible to prevent the development of hepatorenal syndrome (see Chapter 6 for more information on adverse reactions).

Step 2: Drug information

Having identified which aspects of the drug's pharmacology, pharmacokinetics and pharmacodynamics you need to consider, you can refer to the back of the *aide mémoire* to review the relevant drug considerations in more detail.

Pharmacokinetics (see Chapter 5 for more information)

You may be able to focus on specific elements of pharmacokinetics, as not all sections will be relevant to your patient.

Absorption

- Is the drug lipid soluble (absorption may be reduced if cholestasis is present)?
- Absorption may be reduced by ascites, causing an oedematous gut wall. This is not measurable or predictable, so use the normal dose and monitor for efficacy.

Distribution

- Is the drug distributed into water (may be affected by ascites) or fat (may be affected by failure to thrive or cachexia)?
- Is it highly protein bound? More than 80% may be affected by albumin levels <30 g/L.
- Does it displace or is it displaced by bilirubin? It may be affected by high bilirubin levels or may increase the risk of kernicterus in newborns.

Metabolism

- Does the drug have a high extraction ratio (>0.7) such that bioavailability may be affected by portal hypertension/varices causing reduced or absent first-pass metabolism?
- Is the metabolism hepatocyte dependent, i.e. with a low extraction ratio (<0.3) which may be affected by cirrhosis where hepatocyte mass is reduced?
- Is it a prodrug relying on metabolism to be activated?
- Is it metabolised by cytochrome enzymes which may be impaired in cirrhosis?
- Are the metabolites active? If they are, then their clearance must be considered too.
- Are there any genetic factors that may affect metabolism?

Elimination

- Is the drug cleared by biliary excretion? Exclusively or partially?
- Do alternative mechanisms compensate if clearance by one route is impaired?
- Does the drug undergo enterohepatic circulation (may add to any problems with metabolism, and may be impaired if biliary excretion is reduced)?

Side effects

These need to be considered in light of the patient's current and potential problems, for example, a decompensated cirrhotic may not have any signs of renal impairment but the use of a renally toxic drug may increase the risk of developing hepatorenal syndrome. See Chapter 6 for more information on side effects.

Clinical studies

It is also worth considering published clinical studies or articles. You need to be precise about the liver disease and degree of dysfunction your patient exhibits, and be wary of extrapolating data. You should also be cautious about accepting generalisations made in conclusions.

Conclusions

Finally, do not forget to consider all of the non-liver-related factors about your patient – contraindications to therapy, concomitant disease, age, etc. At the end of this process you should be able to come to some sort of conclusion about the use of a specific drug in your patient. It is often not a definitive answer but an educated guess based on the available evidence. At the very least you should be able to give advice to reduce the risks of side effects and provide guidance on the relevant monitoring parameters.

Patient 3 Patient Information
Name/DoB/unit number: Edward Farrell, 15 years
Diagnosis (type/cause) (if known): Thioguanine-induced liver disease
Relevant biochemical tests:

Test	Result – recent changes ↑ ↓ ↔	Normal range
ALT/AST	18 ↔	<60 IU/L
Bilirubin	16 ↔	5–21 µmol/L
Split bilirubin*	N/A	
Alk phos	339 ↔	230–600 IU/L
GGT	9 ↔	<40 IU/L
Albumin	44 ↔	34–48 g/L
INR/PT	1.3 ↔	0.9–1.2
Creatinine/creatinine clearance/GFR**	67 ↔	55–105 µmol/L

Caution: Check for non-liver causes of abnormal results, e.g. warfarin, bone disease.
* May be useful in determining reason for hyperbilirubinaemia – not a routine test.
** Caution with interpreting in cirrhotic patients.

Signs of liver disease and useful test results likely to have an impact on drug handling

Sign	Present?	Tests	Result
Gynaecomastia		Biopsy	Mild fibrosis
Ascites		ERCP/HIDA	
Varices	✓	Ultrasound scan – Doppler	Splenomegaly, nodular liver
Failure to thrive/ wt loss	✓	Endoscopy	Grade 1 varices
Pale stools		MELD/PELD/ Child–Pugh	
Encephalopathy		Encephalopathy score/grade	

Using all the information available, including the signs and test results, tick which apply with severity or grade if known

Effect on kinetics/dynamics		Risk factors for side effects	
Ascites (A/D)		Varices	✓
Cholestasis (A/E)		Coagulopathy or low platelets	Plts 80
Low albumin (D)		Encephalopathy	
Portal hypertension (M)	✓	Pruritus	
Acute liver failure (M)		Alcoholism	
Cirrhosis – compensated (M)		Ascites	
Cirrhosis – decompensated (M)		Renal impairment/hepatorenal	
Encephalopathy (P)		Cirrhosis	

A = absorption; D = distribution; M = metabolism; E = elimination; P = pharmacodynamics.

Drug considerations

Drug: Minocycline

Pharmacokinetics

		Considerations
Absorption		Lipid solubility (absorption affected by ascites)
Distribution		Water/fat Protein binding % Displaced by bilirubin or displaces bilirubin
Metabolism	5% metabolised by the liver	First-pass effect Hepatocyte dependent Prodrug CYPs Active metabolites Genetics
Elimination	60% excreted unchanged in urine 40% biliary excretion	Biliary excretion Alternative mechanisms Enterohepatic recirculation (renal impairment)

Side effects
Consider: GI ulceration, sedation, coagulopathy, platelet effects, effects on fluid balance, effect on electrolytes, biliary sludging, renal impairment, constipation
Oesophagitis/oesophageal ulceration if taken before bed or with inadequate fluids

Hepatoxicity – known hepatotoxin/type
Well known – causes fatty liver, jaundice and transient increases in LFTs

Published information in specific liver diseases/clinical studies
BNF/SPC
BNF – tetracyclines – avoid (or use with caution)
SPC – care should be exercised in administering tetracyclines to patients with hepatic impairment

Concomitant drug interactions and other patient considerations, e.g. age, renal function, contraindications
No other drugs or contraindications

Summary/answer
Hepatotoxicity no more likely in this patient than in someone with normal liver function, therefore no additional concern. Careful counselling required about taking the tablets with plenty of water and remaining upright to avoid oesophageal irritation and risk of oesophagitis/bleeding.

The last example is of a boy who wants to start minocycline for acne, having already tried a variety of topical treatments. His liver disease is mild, and although he has varices he does not need treatment for them and just has a check endoscopy once a year. He is slightly thin, which may be related to his liver disease causing increased calorie requirements, but he is not cholestatic. Minocycline is metabolised by the liver to a very small degree and is mostly excreted unchanged in urine, with 40% cleared by biliary excretion. His liver's metabolising capacity can be assumed to be completely normal, and so you would not expect any changes in the pharmacokinetics of minocycline. The side effect profile is more concerning, as he has varices and minocycline has been reported to cause oesophagitis, which could increase the risk of a variceal bleed. However, with a lot of counselling about how to take the drug (sitting up with plenty of water), the risks are likely to be low and outweighed by the benefits.

Reference

1.   Mehta DK (ed) (2007) *British National Formulary*. No. 53. London: British Medical Association and the Royal Pharmaceutical Society of Great Britain.

9

Scenario 1: Choice of analgesic

Janet Tweed, Faye Croxen, Kylies Foot

When choosing an appropriate analgesic for a patient with liver impairment it is important to first consider the principles of pain management, as you would in any patient. This includes assessing the type of pain, involving the patient in discussion of treatment choices, using pain scores, and using the analgesic ladder to ensure the rational titration of treatment.

This chapter concentrates on some drug choices in acute rather than chronic pain, but the same principles can be used to determine the appropriateness of other types of analgesic. The drugs considered in this section are paracetamol, non-steroidal anti-inflammatories (NSAIDs: specifically diclofenac, ibuprofen, indometacin, naproxen, sulindac and tenoxicam) and opioids (codeine, dihydrocodeine, morphine, pethidine and tramadol). Unless otherwise stated, all pharmacokinetic data originate from standard reference sources [1–5] and apply to adults only.

PARACETAMOL

Summary

Most studies investigating paracetamol pharmacokinetics in patients with liver disease used single doses only. A 50% reduction in clearance and a corresponding increase in half-life have been seen in severe acute hepatitis, the longest half-life being seen in patients with a raised pro-thrombin time (PT). It may therefore be prudent to extend the dose interval in these patients. Cirrhotic patients with a low albumin and a raised PT were also noted to have a prolonged paracetamol half-life, although no accumulation or hepatotoxicity was observed when normal therapeutic doses were administered to these patients for up to five days. In contrast, cirrhotic patients with normal albumin and PT demonstrated no difference in paracetamol pharmacokinetics following single doses, compared to controls. Normal doses of paracetamol can therefore be used in cirrhotic patients requiring short courses.

There is a theoretical concern that chronic alcoholics are at an increased risk of paracetamol hepatotoxicity. However, from the short-term data available in controlled situations, there seems to be no increased risk of hepatotoxicity when these patients are administered therapeutic doses of paracetamol. Some evidence suggests that the potential increased risk of hepatotoxicity may be related more to poor diet and fasting than to the effects of the alcohol. Longer-term controlled studies are still needed to assess the risks of chronic therapeutic dosing in alcoholics.

The evidence suggests that paracetamol is safe to use in the majority of patients with liver disease, with no increased risk of hepatotoxicity when normal doses are used.

Pharmacokinetics of paracetamol

See Table 9.1 for a summary of pharmacokinetic information about paracetamol.

Table 9.1 Pharmacokinetics of paracetamol in adults

Oral bioavailability	80%
Protein binding	<20% at usual therapeutic concentrations (increases with higher concentrations, e.g. overdose)
Half-life	1.5–3 hours
Excreted unchanged in urine	Up to 5%
Biliary excretion of active forms	Minimal
Metabolic pathway	Glucuronidation and sulphation (90%), oxidation (5%) – CYP2E1 (mostly), CYP1A2 and 3A4
	First-pass metabolism of 20%
Active metabolites	Hepatotoxic metabolite (NAPQI)

Absorption

- Paracetamol is readily absorbed from the gastrointestinal tract, peak plasma concentrations occurring 15 minutes to two hours after ingestion.

- Oral bioavailability is approximately 80% and is independent of dose in the range 5–20 mg/kg.

Metabolism

- The majority of paracetamol is conjugated by the liver (to sulphate or glucuronide – approximately 90%) and the remainder is oxidised by cytochrome enzymes (approximately 5%) or excreted unchanged.
- Oxidation is primarily by CYP2E1 to N-acetyl-para-benzoquinoneimine (NAPQI), a highly reactive metabolite, which is then inactivated by reacting with the sulfhydryl groups in glutathione to form mercapturic and cysteine acid conjugates (Figure 9.1).

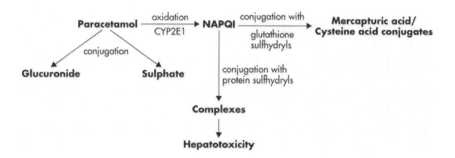

Figure 9.1   Metabolic pathway of paracetamol.

- In paracetamol overdose the pathway producing glucuronide and sulphate conjugates is rapidly overwhelmed and a higher proportion of paracetamol is oxidised to NAPQI. Glutathione stores are swiftly depleted, causing hepatocellular toxicity as the NAPQI reacts with sulfhydryl groups in hepatic proteins rather than glutathione sulfhydryls [6].
- Glutathione depletion can occur in malnourished people and alcoholics.
- The dominant metabolic pathway in neonates and children is sulphate conjugation. Glucuronide conjugation matures more slowly (the urinary glucuronide to sulphate ratio increases throughout childhood from 0.4 in neonates to 2 in adults) [7].
- Children under six years of age seem to be less susceptible to paracetamol toxicity, possibly owing to a more efficient detoxification pathway or greater glutathione content, or simply a greater liver size in relation to body mass [8].

Elimination

- Glucuronide and sulphate conjugates, and the cysteine and mercapturic acid conjugates (formed from inactivation of NAPQI by glutathione), are excreted in the urine.
- Approximately 2–5% of paracetamol is excreted in the urine unchanged.

Some relevant adverse effects

Paracetamol is relatively free of adverse effects, but can cause hepatotoxicity in overdose.

Hepatotoxicity

Hypersensitivity

On rare occasions therapeutic doses of paracetamol have been reported to cause hepatotoxicity as a result of hypersensitivity. Rechallenge with small doses triggered a recurrence of the reaction [9].

Short-term use at therapeutic doses

A daily intake of 4 g paracetamol for a period of two weeks has been shown to cause transient elevations of ALT (more than three times the upper limit of normal) in some healthy adults. All significant ALT elevations resolved after treatment was stopped, and all subjects remained asymptomatic throughout. It has been speculated that prior treatment with paracetamol may desensitise the liver and reduce the likelihood of subsequent elevations of ALT on retreatment. This could account for the generally normal transaminase levels seen in most patient populations compared to the healthy subjects in this trial. The clinical significance of this rise in ALT is unclear, but therapeutic paracetamol ingestion could be considered as a potential cause of elevated ALT in the absence of other causes [10].

Chronic use at therapeutic doses

Isolated cases of chronic paracetamol toxicity have been reported, such as hepatocellular necrosis, hepatic inflammation and fibrosis. These cases occurred in patients taking 2–6 g of paracetamol daily for months or years. In most cases, recovery was prompt when paracetamol was stopped [11, 12].

Acute overdose

Hepatotoxicity from paracetamol overdose can occur with single doses as low as 10–15 g. The risk factors for hepatotoxicity in excessive doses include: induction of cytochrome P450 enzymes; malnutrition or fasting, due to reduced glutathione stores and reduced glucuronidation; chronic alcohol use; and age over five years [8, 13].

Hepatotoxicity in alcoholics

See section on Interactions for mechanism.

Therapeutic doses of paracetamol in alcoholics

There is an abundance of anecdotal reports of the therapeutic use of paracetamol in alcoholics causing greater hepatotoxicity than would normally be expected. These reports have led to the belief that patients who chronically consume alcohol (regardless of whether or not they have liver disease) are at increased risk of developing severe hepatotoxicity from paracetamol. However, in many of the case reports where 'therapeutic' use of paracetamol was reported to cause hepatotoxicity, the dose was often unsubstantiated or underestimated by patients [14]. Other studies have suggested that the increased risk of hepatotoxicity in such patients may be related more to poor diet and fasting than to the effects of the alcohol [15]. Some texts recommend giving ≤2 g/day of paracetamol to patients who drink more than six units of alcohol per day (60 g of ethanol) [16]. However, the available evidence suggests that dose reduction in alcoholics is unnecessary, although caution should be used in those who are concomitantly malnourished.

Acute overdose in alcoholics

There is no good evidence that alcoholics are more susceptible to hepatotoxicity as a result of their alcohol intake. Several large retrospective studies examining hundreds of paracetamol overdoses have shown no difference in hepatotoxicity/survival rate in those who chronically consume alcohol compared to moderate or non-drinkers [14, 17]. However, alcoholics are more likely to present later and to be malnourished, and thus may appear to be more susceptible to paracetamol hepatotoxicity [14].

Haematological effects

There have been isolated reports of thrombocytopenia with paracetamol [2].

Some relevant drug interactions

There are few clinically significant drug interactions with paracetamol.

Inducers of CYP2E1, 1A2 or 3A4, e.g. rifampicin, phenytoin, carbamazepine, phenobarbital

Theoretically these drugs could increase the metabolism of paracetamol to NAPQI, and could increase the risk of hepatotoxicity.

Despite case reports of hepatotoxicity in patients taking enzyme inducers and paracetamol concomitantly, there is currently no good evidence that the interactions are clinically significant when recommended doses of paracetamol are used [5]. However, because of the theoretical basis and the potentially severe outcome, patients taking enzyme-inducing drugs are treated with N-acetylcysteine at a reduced threshold in the event of paracetamol overdose.

Alcohol

The interaction with paracetamol is complex.

Acute alcohol administration

When administered acutely, ethanol competes with paracetamol for CYP2E1 and blocks the active site, theoretically resulting in less formation of NAPQI. The protective, competitive influence of ethanol is thought to be present for as long as alcohol is present in the body [14, 18].

Chronic alcohol administration

With chronic alcohol consumption CYP2E1 is induced, resulting in increased formation of NAPQI. Most of the evidence for this interaction has come from animal studies. Studies in humans indicate only modest, variable and short-lived (five to ten days) induction of CYP2E1 by alcohol [14]. Chronic alcoholics are theoretically at an increased risk of paracetamol hepatotoxicity during the first few days of withdrawal because the competition for CYP2E1 is lost but CYP2E1 remains induced. However, in a number of studies, maximal therapeutic doses given during this time have had no significant adverse effects on LFTs or increases in NAPQI formation [14, 19]. The issue is further complicated by the development of liver damage in alcoholics, which could reduce the metabolising capacity of the liver, thereby offsetting the enzyme induction.

Owing to the theoretical risk of greater NAPQI formation when paracetamol is taken in overdose by alcoholics, they are administered N-acetylcysteine at a reduced threshold.

Isoniazid

As with alcohol, there is a complex interaction between isoniazid and paracetamol, affecting the risk of hepatotoxicity [5].

Clinical studies

As with most medications, no robust assessment of the use of paracetamol in liver disease has been performed, although small studies of paracetamol metabolism in various forms of liver disease have been undertaken. Although limited, the results of some of these studies are summarised below.

The half-life of paracetamol has been shown to be prolonged during acute viral hepatitis and in patients with severe chronic liver disease. Most studies were single-dose studies. One study looked at the pharmacokinetics of paracetamol (1 g) in ten patients with acute viral hepatitis (ALT increased at least tenfold and acute onset of symptoms) and 20 controls. In the hepatitis patients the paracetamol dose was given in both the acute phase and in the convalescence phase (approximately one month after complete biochemical recovery). At the time of the acute attack, peak concentrations of paracetamol did not differ significantly compared to the recovery phase, nor to the 20 controls. However, during acute hepatitis the half-life of paracetamol was significantly increased compared to the convalescent phase (3.2 h vs 2.3 h), as a result of a 50% reduction in clearance. The longest half-lives were seen in those with raised prothrombin time (PT). The authors concluded that normal dose paracetamol with an extended dosage interval should be given in serious cases of acute viral hepatitis where PT is prolonged [20].

Other studies have also demonstrated similar increases in half-life when comparing paracetamol pharmacokinetics in patients with decompensated chronic liver disease to normal subjects. Patients with cirrhosis who have a normal plasma albumin concentration and PT have been shown to have a similar paracetamol half-life and clearance to those of healthy subjects. However, cirrhotic patients with a low plasma albumin and an increased PT were found to have a prolonged paracetamol half-life. Despite this, no accumulation and no evidence of hepatotoxicity was demonstrated when therapeutic doses of paracetamol were given to patients with decompensated liver diseases for three to five days [21].

Studies of drug use in paediatric patients are infrequently performed. In one small study, the metabolism of a single dose of paracetamol (10 mg/kg) was assessed in 13 children with liver disease between the ages of seven months and 12 years. No significant differences were found in comparison to previously reported results in healthy children of similar ages, but there was a trend to increasing half-life in the more severely ill patients. Unfortunately, interpretation of these results is difficult, as the patient group was small and heterogeneous, spanning a large age range and having a substantial variation in the severity of liver disease, with only four of the 13 patients having a PT of more than 15 seconds. There was also no control group [7].

One study looked at the proportion of paracetamol that was converted to NAPQI in 19 patients with hepatocellular carcinoma, 39 with chronic hepatitis B and 26 healthy controls. The excretion of mercapturic acid and cysteine conjugates in urine was used as an indirect measurement of NAPQI formation. Compared to the other groups, the formation of these conjugates in those with hepatocellular carcinoma was significantly increased (by approximately two and a half times), whereas the levels of glucuronide conjugate were significantly reduced [22].

NSAIDS

Summary

Irrespective of the pharmacokinetics of NSAIDs in patients with liver disease, the risks of adverse effects will outweigh the benefits of treatment in many patients. Side effects of note are gastrointestinal bleeding, reduction in glomerular filtration rate (GFR), inhibition of platelet aggregation, and oedema and electrolyte abnormalities. Data are available suggesting that ibuprofen has the lowest risk of bleeding and sulindac may be safer for the kidneys (the latter has been disputed). However, despite this, all NSAIDs should be avoided in patients with fibrosis, cirrhosis or acute liver failure, in whom the risks of variceal bleeding, hepatorenal syndrome, encephalopathy, etc. are too great. Even if the Summary of Product Characteristics for an NSAID does not explicitly contraindicate or caution against use in these types of patient, the undesirable or adverse effects may preclude its use.

Although reliable pharmacokinetic study data are lacking, analysis of basic pharmacokinetic information suggests that NSAIDs may be considered as possible treatments for patients with non-cirrhotic, non-fibrotic liver conditions such as hepatitis or cholestasis. NSAID toxicity due to changes in plasma levels may nevertheless occur. For example, because most NSAIDs are highly protein bound, high bilirubin levels could increase the free fraction available (although this increased unbound fraction is also more available for metabolism in the liver, provided the liver is capable); cholestasis may reduce the elimination of the NSAIDs excreted in bile (indometacin and sulindac). Cholestasis may also theoretically reduce or delay the absorption of fat-soluble NSAIDs such as ibuprofen. Delayed absorption has been noted in single-dose studies with naproxen.

Hepatotoxicity is an extremely rare but unpredictable side effect associated with most NSAIDs. There is some suggestion that diclofenac and sulindac have the highest risk, whereas ibuprofen has the lowest risk.

Pharmacokinetics

See Table 9.2 for a summary of NSAID pharmacokinetic information.

Absorption

* Most NSAIDs are well absorbed from the gastrointestinal tract, although there can be substantial inter- and intra-individual variations, e.g. indometacin [1, 24].
* The presence of cholestasis may theoretically reduce the oral absorption of the more lipid-soluble NSAIDs, such as ibuprofen.

Table 9.2 Pharmacokinetics of NSAIDs in adults

Drug	Oral bioavailability (%)	Protein binding (%)	Half-life (hours)	% excreted unchanged in urine	Biliary excretion of active forms	Metabolic pathway	Active metabolites
Diclofenac	50	>99	1–2	<1	Negligible, if at all	Extensive in liver – CYP2C9 – hydroxylation then sulphation/glucuronidation. First-pass metabolism of 50%	4- and possibly 3-hydroxydiclofenac but negligible anti-inflammatory activity compared to diclofenac
Ibuprofen	71*	99	2	<10	No	Extensive in liver CYP2C9 – hydroxylation followed by conjugation and oxidation	No
Indometacin	Almost 100	90–99	1–16 mean 4	5–20	Yes and enterohepatic circulation	Extensive in liver – glucuronidation, demethylation and deacylation	No

Table 9.2 Continued

Drug	Oral bioavailability (%)	Protein binding (%)	Half-life (hours)	% excreted unchanged in urine	Biliary excretion of active forms	Metabolic pathway	Active metabolites
Naproxen	95	>99 (decreases at higher plasma concentrations)	12–15	<10	No information [23]	Extensive in liver – CYP2C9 Demethylation and glucuronidation	No
Sulindac	90	93 (and high for metabolites)	7–8 (16.4 sulfide)	<1% of sulindac dose appears as active sulfide metabolite	Yes; sulindac and sulfone undergo extensive enterohepatic circulation relative to sulfide	Extensive in liver – oxidation to sulfone, reduction to sulfide and glucuronidation	Sulindac sulfide (parent is prodrug)
Tenoxicam	100	>99	44–100 mean 72	<0.5%	No	Extensive in liver – CYP2C9 oxidation and conjugation	No

*71% bioavailability of the S-enantiomer is produced by racemic ibuprofen. The S-enantiomer is the active form.

Distribution

- As the protein binding of most NSAIDs is very high, raised bilirubin and/or low albumin levels could increase the free fraction of NSAIDs available for pharmacological activity.

Metabolism

- Most NSAIDs are metabolised in the liver to inactive metabolites.
- Diclofenac undergoes presystemic metabolism, and administration via the rectal route will avoid this first-pass effect. This may be beneficial in patients who have significantly impaired metabolic capacity, where peak plasma levels may otherwise be raised if the oral route is used.
- Sulindac is an inactive prodrug which needs to be converted in the liver to its active metabolite, sulindac sulfide. The metabolic pathway for sulindac is complicated, even in healthy subjects, by the reversibility of this process, the possibility of conversion to an inactive sulfone metabolite, and the extensive enterohepatic circulation of all three species [25, 26].
- In general, it has been shown that the plasma concentrations of NSAIDs are elevated when administered to patients with significant hepatic impairment (see Clinical studies section for details).

Elimination

- Most NSAIDs are metabolised in the liver, with the metabolites being excreted in the urine. The amount of each NSAID excreted unchanged in the urine is generally very small, the main exception being indometacin.
- The half-lives of NSAIDs vary widely. In liver disease, drugs with shorter half-lives are preferred, as those with long half-lives are more prone to accumulation.
- Indometacin and sulindac undergo enterohepatic circulation.

Some relevant adverse effects

Hepatotoxicity

Hepatotoxicity is an extremely rare but unpredictable side effect associated with most NSAIDs, including those that are COX-2 selective [27].

Risk factors have been discussed in a number of sources, although opinions vary. Controversial risk factors include gender, age, the presence of underlying autoimmune disease and chemical structure [27–30]. Some authors state that there is no clear link between the structure of an NSAID and the likelihood of developing hepatic injury [29]; others suggest that these adverse reactions are more frequently reported with pyrazolone, indole and propionic acid derivatives than with fenamates and oxicams [26]. There is also some suggestion that hepatotoxicity is more common with diclofenac and sulindac [4, 27, 28], whereas ibuprofen has the lowest risk [4]. Additionally, users of NSAIDs for rheumatoid arthritis have been shown to have an increased risk compared to those being treated for osteoarthritis; concomitant exposure to other hepatotoxic drugs may be another risk factor [28]. NSAID-induced hepatotoxicity is not generally dose related [12, 29].

Although NSAID-induced hepatotoxicity can occur at any time, it usually occurs within six to 12 weeks of the start of treatment [28]. Effects range from asymptomatic rises in LFTs to, rarely, fulminant hepatic necrosis resulting in death or the need for transplantation [30]. Mortality has been estimated at <1/100 000 patient-years of exposure [30], whereas borderline, frequently transient, increases in one or more LFTs have been reported in up to 15% of patients in clinical trials [4]. The presenting pattern can be hepatocellular or cholestatic [30], and the range of hepatotoxic reactions reported include cholestasis, hepatitis, cholestatic hepatitis, hepatonecrotic lesions, fulminant hepatic necrosis and hepatic failure [12, 29]. More details regarding specific hepatotoxicity, onset, clinical features, prognosis, etc. for individual NSAIDs can be found in the published literature.

The mechanism for most NSAID-induced hepatotoxic reactions is idiosyncratic, either immunological (hypersensitivity) or metabolic in type [29].

Given the potential hepatotoxicity of NSAIDs, some have suggested that raised transaminase levels are an early indicator of reversible liver toxicity during prolonged NSAID courses, and therefore should be monitored reasonably closely [31]. However, it should be noted that minor subclinical abnormalities in LFTs rarely represent acute liver injury [32, 33].

Gastrointestinal effects

NSAIDs are well known for causing upper gastrointestinal ulceration and haemorrhage [4]. Ibuprofen (<1600 mg/day) is associated with the lowest risk [2, 34].

A case–control study in cirrhotic patients with portal hypertension and varices concluded that patients who use NSAIDs are about three times more likely to have a first variceal bleeding episode than those who do not. The risk appeared to be mainly due to aspirin, either alone or in combination with other NSAIDs, and only in patients with moderate or severe varices. No conclusion could be drawn as to whether exclusive use of non-aspirin NSAIDs increased the risk. The majority of patients who used aspirin were taking 300 mg or more a day. The authors discuss the possible mechanisms, which include the inhibitory effect of aspirin on platelets [27].

Haematological effects

NSAIDs can reversibly inhibit platelet aggregation and may prolong bleeding time, but only for as long as the drug remains in the system. Significant bleeding complications generally only occur in patients with previous coagulopathy problems, such as haemophiliacs or patients with liver disease. Some NSAIDs are more potent inhibitors of platelet function than others, and it has been suggested that, based on this consideration and a short half-life, ibuprofen may be one of the better options in these patients [4].

In addition, there are occasional reports of NSAIDs causing thrombocytopenia, which, although symptomatic, is generally mild and reversible on discontinuation of the drug [4, 27].

Endocrine/metabolic effects

Oedema and electrolyte abnormalities have been reported with NSAIDs [4, 27].

Renal effects

NSAIDs inhibit prostaglandin synthesis, and in so doing can reduce GFR in susceptible patients, including those with cirrhosis. A number of renal complications can occur, including acute renal failure. All NSAIDs have been associated with nephrotoxicity. There is a small amount of data suggesting that renal effects are less likely to occur with sulindac, but studies relate to short-term therapy only, and there have been case reports of acute renal failure developing in high-risk patients [4, 27, 35].

Various NSAIDs have been shown to reduce GFR in patients with cirrhosis. Decompensated cirrhotic patients with ascites have the highest risk [35, 36].

Some relevant drug interactions

NSAIDs metabolised by CYP2C9 (ibuprofen, diclofenac, naproxen and tenoxicam)

CYP2C9 inhibitors could theoretically increase plasma levels of these NSAIDs, and similarly enzyme inducers may reduce plasma levels [5].

Interaction with diuretics

Renal prostaglandins are involved in the mechanism of action of diuretics. NSAIDs block the synthesis of prostaglandins and hence can reduce the effects of diuretics. The combination may also increase the risk of NSAID-induced nephrotoxicity [5]. Patients with cirrhosis and ascites are at a greater risk of this interaction.

Clinical studies

There are few, if any, noteworthy studies of NSAID use in liver disease. This is because they are rarely used in liver disease because of their adverse effect profile. Most studies conducted used a single dose only, thus neglecting to assess the effects of multiple doses that are used in real-life scenarios.

Pharmacokinetics in liver impairment

Diclofenac

A small open-labelled study evaluated the pharmacokinetics of a single 150 mg oral dose of diclofenac in six healthy subjects with normal liver function, six patients with chronic active hepatitis and six patients with alcoholic cirrhosis. Few baseline characteristics were provided, but the cirrhotic patients had a significantly higher Child–Pugh score and lower albumin than patients with hepatitis. The pharmacokinetics were generally similar in healthy patients and those with hepatitis, but the AUC for diclofenac and its 4-hydroxy metabolite were around three times higher in the cirrhotic patients. In addition, the half-life of diclofenac was approximately 1.7 times longer and Cmax was approximately doubled in cirrhotics. This study indicates that if a single dose of diclofenac is to be used in cirrhotics, one third of the usual dose should be given [37].

Novartis Pharmaceuticals, the manufacturers of Voltarol®, state that 'In patients with chronic hepatitis or non-decompensated cirrhosis, the kinetics and metabolism of diclofenac are the same as in patients without liver disease' [38].

Ibuprofen

In a single-dose study examining the pharmacokinetics of sulindac and ibuprofen in 15 patients with alcoholic liver disease, no statistically significant effects were noted for ibuprofen elimination, half-life or AUC compared to the controls. However, there appeared to be delayed absorption in some patients [25].

A later single-dose study in eight patients with moderate to severe cirrhosis and a PT of 2–5 seconds above the upper limit of normal, showed an approximate doubling of the half-life compared to controls. Metabolic inversion of the inactive R-ibuprofen to the active S-ibuprofen may also be impaired in hepatic cirrhosis, because the AUC ratio of R- to S-ibuprofen was significantly higher in patients with cirrhosis. Medicinal ibuprofen is supplied as a racemic mixture [39].

Naproxen

Pharmacokinetics were assessed in ten patients with alcoholic cirrhosis (average age 46) and ten healthy individuals (average age 29). Single-dose pharmacokinetics after a 375 mg dose, and steady-state pharmacokinetics after 13 doses of 375 mg twice daily were examined. The percentage of unbound naproxen (determining the pharmacological effect) was found to increase in the cirrhotic patients, possibly due to the raised bilirubin levels and/or low albumin. Clearance of unbound drug at steady state was reduced by approximately 60% in the patients with liver disease, leading the authors to recommend at least halving the dose of naproxen if it is to be used in patients with chronic alcoholic liver disease. A significantly younger control group may have influenced the results [40].

In another trial the pharmacokinetics of a single dose of naproxen was studied in 11 patients with liver disease (four severe hepatitis with cholestasis; two extrahepatic cholestasis; one chronic alcoholic cirrhosis; two active chronic hepatitis, with and without symptoms; one asymptomatic PBC; and one asymptomatic hepatic cirrhosis). In two of the seven patients with cholestasis, a significant delay in absorption occurred. In most of the patients studied there was a significant decrease in elimination, increasing the half-life from around 14 hours to 20 hours [41].

Sulindac

In a single-dose study in patients with alcoholic liver disease (divided into fair or poor hepatic function) the activation of sulindac was delayed, and plasma concentration of the active sulfide metabolite was maximal about eight hours after an oral dose, compared to approximately two hours in healthy subjects. In addition, compared to controls, the AUC for the active metabolite was four times higher in those with the poorest hepatic function and almost double in those with fair hepatic function [25].

Tenoxicam

Tenoxicam protein binding has been shown in single-dose studies to be unrelated to the plasma concentration of albumin; however, patients with cirrhosis and very high plasma bilirubin levels (100–200 µmol/L) have demonstrated a significant increase in the unbound concentration of tenoxicam [42].

A single-dose pharmacokinetic study was performed using tenoxicam 20 mg in six patients with compensated cirrhosis. Compared to healthy subjects, no differences in pharmacokinetics were seen [43].

Potential benefits of NSAIDs in some liver disorders

In certain liver disorders NSAIDs may actually be of benefit. For example, in biliary colic there is no impairment of liver synthetic function and thus NSAIDs may be safe to use. Prostaglandins are thought to increase pressure, secretions and contractions of the gallbladder, and thus there is a theoretical basis for pain improvement with NSAIDs. Studies with diclofenac have also demonstrated a reduced occurrence of cholecystitis, a frequent complication of biliary colic [2, 4, 44].

OPIOIDS

Summary

The pharmacokinetics, pharmacodynamics and adverse effect profile of opioid analgesics are all relevant when considering the risks involved in using these drugs in patients with liver disease. There are also small variations between drugs in relation to pharmacokinetics and side effects, which may affect choice in certain circumstances. The decision to use opioids, the choice of opioid and the dose will therefore depend significantly on the type and extent of liver disease, and the signs and symptoms the patient displays or is prone to developing.

Most opioids are metabolised in the liver and have a high intrinsic clearance/high first-pass effect. Therefore, when liver metabolism is impaired or when there is decreased blood flow through the liver (e.g. cirrhosis), clearance of opioids may be reduced, resulting in a prolonged duration of action and possible toxicity. Portal hypertension may also increase the oral bioavailability and hence the toxicity risk of opioids, as first-pass metabolism will be reduced. The probability of toxicity occurring is additionally dependent on a number of other patient and drug-related factors.

Example of factors which could decrease opioid levels are:

- The presence of ascites may reduce oral absorption.
- Distribution of water-soluble drugs into ascitic fluid may reduce the amount available for circulation.
- Impaired metabolic capacity may decrease the conversion of drugs to active metabolites, e.g. codeine, tramadol.

Example of factors that could increase opioid effects:

- The effects of fat-soluble drugs may be increased in cachectic patients.
- Cholestasis may reduce the elimination of morphine and codeine through bile.
- Opioid receptor sensitivity may be enhanced in liver disease.

Because of these many confounding factors, it is hard to predict the pharmacokinetics of opioids in patients with liver disease.

The sedative effects of opioids are dose related, and this should be taken into account when using them in patients who may decompensate and become encephalopathic. It is important that opioids are started at low doses in these patients. In addition, opioids often cause constipation, which could precipitate hepatic encephalopathy.

In patients with alcoholic liver disease who are prone to alcoholic seizures, it is best to avoid pethidine and tramadol because of their epileptogenic potential.

Other side effects which may be of concern in some patients are oedema and pruritus. There are very few reports of hepatic injury with opioids.

Opioids with long half-lives, such as pethidine, or slow-release preparations should generally be avoided, as if toxicity does ensue it will be prolonged. However, after continued unproblematic use of a regular opioid dose a slow-release preparation may be tried cautiously in patients with stable liver disease.

Clinical studies in patients with liver disease are lacking. Those that are published reveal wide inter-individual variability in pharmacokinetic parameters between patients, and consequently interpretation of the data is difficult.

A limited number of small single-dose studies have demonstrated that morphine metabolism is impaired in patients with decompensated cirrhosis, and half-life can be doubled. Information on multiple morphine doses in cirrhotic patients is lacking, but because of the demonstrated prolonged half-life in single-dose studies, accumulation could occur, and an increased dosing interval of approximately twofold is recommended in some reports.

Cirrhotic patients and those with acute viral hepatitis have experienced a doubling of the half-life of pethidine and a corresponding reduction in clearance compared to healthy subjects.

There is a scarcity of information regarding use of codeine, dihydrocodeine and tramadol in patients with liver impairment. On the basis of pharmacokinetic properties, dihydrocodeine may be preferred over codeine. Owing to a lack of information and the potentially detrimental characteristics of tramadol, other opioids should be used in preference if possible.

Regardless of whether the pharmacokinetics of a drug is altered or not, the response to sedative drugs may be increased in patients with liver disease, perhaps as a result of increased end-organ sensitivity. Opioids should therefore be used cautiously, ensuring the patient is closely monitored.

Pharmacokinetics

See Table 9.3 for a summary of opioid pharmacokinetic information.

Absorption

- Most opioids used orally are well absorbed from the gastrointestinal tract.
- None of the opioids discussed are highly lipid soluble, therefore the presence of cholestasis is unlikely to affect their oral absorption.

Distribution

- As the protein binding of most opioids is low, alterations in bilirubin and albumin levels are unlikely to increase the free fraction of opioids.

Table 9.3 Pharmacokinetics of opioids in adults

Drug	Oral bioavailability (%)	Protein binding (%)	Half-life (hours)	% excreted unchanged in urine	Biliary excretion of active forms	Metabolic pathway	Active metabolites
Codeine	40–70 [45]	7–25	3–4	6–8	Some	Principal route is glucuronidation to codeine-6-glucuronide. Also demethylation. 5–15% of dose converted to morphine by O-demethylation (CYP2D6) First-pass metabolism of 50%	Yes. Significant part of analgesic effect thought to be due to conversion to morphine
Dihydrocodeine	21	No information [46]	3.4–4.5 mean 4	35	No information [46]	Demethylation and glucuronidation similar to codeine. O-demethylation to dihydromorphine (CYP2D6) Substantial first-pass metabolism	Yes. Dihydromorphine – potent analgesic, but analgesia primarily due to dihydrocodeine

Table 9.3 Continued

Drug	Oral bioavailability (%)	Protein binding (%)	Half-life (hours)	% excreted unchanged in urine	Biliary excretion of active forms	Metabolic pathway	Active metabolites
Morphine	10–50 mean 30	25–30	1–5 mean 3	5–10	Yes and minor enterohepatic circulation	Extensive in liver, mainly as glucuronidation. First pass metabolism of 50–66%	Yes. 5% of dose is converted to morphine-6-glucuronide which is a much more potent analgesic than morphine
Pethidine	Mean 50	40–50	3–6	0.6–27 (pH dependent, less with higher pH)	No information [47]	Extensive in liver via hydrolysis and N-demethylation, followed by partial conjugation. First pass metabolism of 47–61%	Yes. Norpethidine which is half as potent an analgesic, but potent convulsant – causes tremor and seizures Long half-life, up to 20 hours Cleared renally
Tramadol	70% following single dose, 90% at steady state [48]	20	6	30	Not significant [49]	N- and O-demethylation via CYP3A4 and CYP2D6 followed by glucuronidation or sulphation First-pass metabolism of 20–30% [49]	Yes. CYP2D6 O-demethylation produces active metabolite

Metabolism

- Most opioids are metabolised in the liver and many (exceptions include tramadol) undergo a high first-pass effect [50]. Because of this, clearance is highly dependent on liver blood flow, rather than the capability of hepatocyte enzymes. If liver blood flow is reduced, as in hepatic cirrhosis with portal hypertension for example, the metabolism of most opioids would be expected to decrease, with a subsequent increase in oral bioavailability and risk of accumulation.

- Some opioids are available in rectal formulations, and administration via this route avoids the first-pass effect. If liver metabolism is sufficiently impaired, administration via this route would theoretically cause less of an increase in peak opioid levels.

- A significant proportion of the analgesic effect of codeine and tramadol is thought to be due to the hepatic production of active intermediate metabolites. Patients with reduced metabolic capacity may therefore be expected to derive a diminished analgesic effect. However, the clinical significance of this is difficult to predict, since the metabolism of the active metabolite as well as the parent compound will be impaired, leading to reduced clearance of both. The analgesic efficacy of tramadol is further complicated by its multiple mechanisms of action. Although the parent drug has noradrenergic and serotoninergic properties, which are thought to contribute to the analgesic effect, it is the active intermediate metabolite that possesses a much greater affinity for opioid receptors than the parent compound [3, 51].

- Although glucuronidation is thought to be less affected than oxidation in patients with cirrhosis [50], morphine clearance may be reduced and the half-life prolonged [27]. A reduction in first-pass metabolism could increase the bioavailability of oral morphine, but will also reduce the formation of the active (morphine-6-glucuronide) and inactive metabolites. The clinical significance of this is uncertain [50].

Elimination

- Most opioids are metabolised in the liver, the water-soluble conjugates being eliminated renally.
- The majority of opioids have a half life of around 2 to 5 hours.
- The active metabolite of pethidine has a longer half life.
- Drugs with shorter half-lives are usually favoured in liver disease, as any problem encountered can be rapidly reversed. However, the half-life of an opioid is not the only limiting factor with regard to duration of action. The onset and duration of therapeutic effect of a single dose may have more to do with distribution and redistribution of a drug into and out of the brain, a process that is partially affected by a drug's lipophilicity [52].

- Approximately one-third of both dihydrocodeine and tramadol are eliminated by the kidneys. Manufacturer's data for tramadol suggest that in hepatic or renal impairment the increase in half-life should be relatively low as long as one of these organs is functioning normally [48].

Pharmacodynamics

End-organ sensitivity to opioids may be increased in liver disease, in terms of both analgesic properties and adverse effects, meaning that even if the pharmacokinetics of an opioid are not altered, the dose requirement in a patient with liver disease may be less.

Some relevant adverse effects

Hepatotoxicity

There are very few reports of hepatic injury with opioids. Dextropropoxyphene was well known to cause hepatotoxicity, but is no longer marketed in the UK.

- There is one reported case of immunological hepatic injury, thought to be due to pethidine [53].
- There is one published report of unintentional tramadol overdose causing acute fulminant hepatic necrosis and death. The exact amount taken was not known, but may have been more than twice the maximum daily dose of 100 mg four times a day for a period of days. Hepatitis and liver failure are listed as possible adverse effects in some US, but no UK product information [54].

Biliary effects

Morphine can reduce biliary secretions, and patients with biliary colic may experience an exacerbation of pain after morphine. Similarly, opioids such as morphine can cause bile duct spasm [27]. Opioid-induced spasm of the sphincter of Oddi and increased intrabiliary pressure may result in a secondary increase in LFTs [55].

Gastrointestinal effects

All opioids reduce gastrointestinal motility and cause constipation. There is some evidence to suggest that the incidence of constipation is lower with tramadol than with comparable agents for equivalent pain relief [48, 56]. However, it should still be used with caution in suscept-ible patients [56].

Neurological effects

All opioids cause drowsiness and have the potential to precipitate or worsen encephalopathy. Tolerance generally develops with long-term use [2].

Norpethidine, a metabolite of pethidine, can cause tremor and seizures. The risk increases following repeated doses, owing to accumu-lation of the metabolite (longer half-life than pethidine) and resulting high plasma concentrations. Although patients with cirrhosis may have impaired formation of norpethidine, they may still be at increased risk of cumulative toxicity because of the slower elimination of the metab-olite and their increased sensitivity to the effects of opioids [57].

Tramadol lowers the seizure threshold and could also precipitate seizures in susceptible individuals [48], such as alcoholics.

Endocrine/metabolic effects

Opioids have an antidiuretic action and oedema has been reported with several opioids [26].

Dermatological effects

Opioids with histamine-releasing properties can cause itching in some patients. This is thought to be due to opioid effects on neurons as well as histamine release, as itching has also been provoked by opioids that do not release histamine, and is relieved by small doses of naloxone [27].

Some relevant drug interactions

Opioids metabolised by CYP2D6 (codeine, dihydrocodeine, tramadol, and by CYP3A4 tramadol)

CYP2D6 and CYP3A4 inhibitors may increase plasma levels of opioids metabolised by these enzymes, and similarly enzyme inducers may reduce plasma levels. CYP3A4 levels may also be decreased in cirrhosis, further complicating the picture.

Alcohol

Chronic alcohol consumption can induce CYP450 enzymes, whereas acute alcohol intake can inhibit cytochrome P450 enzymes. Prediction of drug handling in alcoholic liver disease is therefore complicated.

Clinical studies

Unfortunately there is a paucity of clinical studies relating to opioid use in hepatically impaired patients. Those that have been performed are small, often involving scarcely more than ten patients, and only using single doses. This may not adequately reveal the cumulative effects of repeat dosing. The inter-individual variability in pharmacokinetic parameters between patients is often great, and clinical trials with small numbers may not be sufficiently large to detect the overall effect. In many cases, larger studies are needed to confirm the findings. Nevertheless, it is still useful to consider the clinical information available in conjunction with the pharmacokinetic theory.

Morphine

Some studies have suggested that the pharmacokinetics of morphine is altered in patients with liver disease, whereas other studies have found no such effect. The conflicting data are likely to be due to variable patient selection.

In one study, no pharmacokinetic differences were noted when a single 0.15 mg/kg intravenous dose was given to six cirrhotic patients and six healthy subjects. However, the cirrhotic patients had no manifestations of end-stage disease, normal prothrombin times and relatively normal liver function tests. Four had experienced prior encephalopathy [58].

In a controlled trial involving eight decompensated cirrhotic patients (compared to six cancer patients with normal liver/kidney function), the half-life of morphine was increased and the clearance was reduced. The differences were statistically significant. Patients in this trial were administered a single dose of 4 mg IV morphine and, on a separate occasion, a single dose of 10 mg oral morphine. All patients had a history of encephalopathy, six had ascites, and two had oesophageal varices. There were many inadequacies in this trial: one patient only received 5 mg oral morphine; one received the IV dose but not the oral dose; one did not receive the IV dose; and the control group was administered 20 mg oral morphine rather than 10 mg [59].

Similarly, another small trial (six healthy subjects and eight alcoholic patients with cirrhosis) demonstrated an approximate doubling of the half-life and halving of clearance in the cirrhotic patients after a single 0.1 mg/kg intravenous dose of morphine. A 1.5–2-fold increase in the administration interval was recommended in order to avoid accumulation [60].

A later study also showed that the half-life of oral morphine approximately doubled in cirrhotic patients compared to controls following a single dose of 30 mg sustained-release morphine. In addition, the peak plasma concentration of morphine was around three times higher in the cirrhotic patients. Changes in pharmacokinetic parameters reached statistical significance. Precise baseline characteristics were not specified in this study, but all 12 patients had oesophageal varices/portal hypertension, none had ascites, and albumin and bilirubin were in the normal range. The cirrhotic patients were said to be over-sedated and experienced more adverse effects than the controls, although none developed encephalopathy [61].

Crotty *et al.* [62] used hepatic vein catheterisation to determine the hepatic extraction of 1 mg IV morphine in eight controls (undergoing heart catheterisation) and eight alcoholic cirrhotic patients with a history of variceal bleeding. The extraction ratio was reduced by 25% in the cirrhotic group. However, bias may have been introduced, as although 11 controls were admitted to the study, three were excluded because their liver blood flow was higher than normal.

Extrahepatic clearance of morphine has been shown to be greater in those with liver impairment. In cirrhotic patients as much as 30% of the morphine may undergo extrahepatic elimination [60, 62]. It is thought that extrahepatic glucuronidation in the intestine, kidney and brain may increase to compensate for the insufficient hepatic metabolism [50].

Overall, clinical trials have shown that the metabolism of single doses of morphine is significantly impaired in patients with decompensated cirrhosis, but possibly not in those with compensated cirrhosis.

Pethidine

Patients with cirrhosis and acute viral hepatitis may have a 50% reduction in pethidine clearance [63, 64]. In a single-dose study, 0.8 mg/kg of pethidine were given intravenously to eight healthy volunteers and ten patients with liver cirrhosis (nine alcohol induced, all with a history of varices and/or ascites). There was an approximate doubling of the half-life and halving of the clearance in the cirrhotic patients, both of which reached statistical significance [63].

Another study using the same dose assessed pharmacokinetic parameters in 15 healthy volunteers and 14 patients with an acute exacerbation of viral hepatitis. None had significantly altered prothrombin times, but all had significantly raised transaminase levels. Similar alterations in pharmacokinetics were observed. Acute viral hepatitis increased the half-life from 3.37 hours to 6.99 hours (p<0.001) (range: 4.4–14.4 hours), and a corresponding halving of clearance was also observed. Five of the hepatitis patients were restudied at least one month after their LFTs returned to normal, at which point half-life and clearance were comparable to control values [64].

One small study showed that five men with hepatic cirrhosis had significantly lower pethidine clearance, greater bioavailability and longer half-life than six healthy subjects. The average half-life was increased from 5.2 hours to 11.4 hours in the cirrhotic group [57].

All three studies maintained alkalinity of urine by administering an agent such as sodium bicarbonate in order to minimise differences in urinary excretion.

Tramadol

Product information for tramadol states that the half-life was increased at least twofold in patients with cirrhosis [48]. It has also been shown that renal excretion of unchanged drug increased to 30% in cirrhotic patients, compared to 10% in healthy patients [50].

Codeine and dihydrocodeine

There is a scarcity of clinical trials regarding use of codeine and dihydrocodeine in liver impairment.

CASE STUDIES

See Appendix 1 for details of the following five patient cases.

Patient 1 – Mild hepatitis without cirrhosis

The synthetic and metabolic capacity of this patient's liver is unlikely to be affected by the isolated rise in ALT and drug handling is unlikely to be altered. It is important to ensure that the patient has no signs of cirrhosis, as many diseases that present with this clinical picture can be cirrhotic despite near-normal laboratory tests.

Paracetamol

- Paracetamol can safely be given to this patient in normal therapeutic doses.
- If this patient was alcoholic or malnourished it might raise additional concerns. Information regarding the therapeutic use of paracetamol in alcoholics is limited and conflicting. Considering the evidence available, current practice is not to reduce the dose of paracetamol in alcoholics. However, if the patient were malnourished a dose reduction might be considered.
- If the patient had acute viral hepatitis with significantly raised transaminases and a raised PT, an increase in the dosage interval of paracetamol should be considered as the clearance of paracetamol has been shown to be reduced by approximately 50% in these types of patients.

Non-steroidal anti-inflammatory drugs (NSAIDs)

- NSAIDs can be used in this patient at normal therapeutic doses.
- Given the rare but potential hepatotoxic risk with NSAIDs, patients should be instructed to be aware of the symptoms of hepatotoxicity and to report fatigue, malaise, anorexia, nausea and vomiting.

Opioids

- Opioids can be used in this patient at normal therapeutic doses.
- If the patient had acute viral hepatitis with significantly raised transaminases, an increase in the dosage interval of pethidine should be considered as the clearance of pethidine has been shown to be reduced by approximately 50% in these types of patients.

Patient 2 – Cholestasis

The synthetic and metabolic capacity of this patient's liver is unlikely to be affected by cholestasis. However, consideration needs to be given to protein binding (the patient has hyperbilirubinaemia); excretion of the drug or metabolites in bile (the patient has cholestasis); and the lipophilicity of the drug (some lipophilic drugs require bile salts for absorption, and these would be reduced in cholestasis).

Paracetamol

Paracetamol can be safely administered to this patient in normal therapeutic doses.

NSAIDs

Many centres prefer to avoid using NSAIDs in any patient with liver
disease because of their side-effect profile. However, if the liver disorder
is purely cholestatic in origin and the disease has not progressed to cirrhosis and portal hypertension, NSAIDs may be an option. Any
risk–benefit assessment should consider the potential risk of hepatotoxicity, albeit rare. There are no specific contraindications in this patient
because they are not cirrhotic, do not have deranged clotting, and are
unlikely to be at increased risk of deteriorating renal function. If deemed
necessary an NSAID could be used cautiously.

It is important to note that other types of patients who are chronically cholestatic may have impaired absorption of vitamin K and a
raised INR. In these types of patients there is an increased risk of bleeding, and NSAIDs should therefore be avoided.

- Cholestasis may reduce the absorption of the highly lipophilic ibuprofen.
- All NSAIDs are highly protein bound and increased levels of free drug
  may occur in the presence of a raised bilirubin, because it can displace the
  bound drug from albumin.
- The metabolism of NSAIDs is unlikely to be affected in this patient.
- Cholestasis may reduce the elimination of certain NSAIDs that are
  excreted via the biliary tract (e.g. sulindac, indometacin).
- Ibuprofen is associated with the lowest risk of GI bleeding compared to
  other NSAIDs.

Taking into account pharmacokinetics, adverse effects and clinical
studies, ibuprofen may be considered the best choice in this patient, for
the following reasons:

- Short half-life
- No biliary excretion of active forms
- Possibly the lowest risk of hepatotoxicity
- Lowest risk of bleeding when used at doses <1600 mg/day.

The possibility of incomplete absorption from the gastrointestinal
tract, because of the highly lipophilic nature of ibuprofen, should be

considered, as should the possibility of increased plasma levels due to high protein binding.

Diclofenac may be a second-line option, but it has a higher risk of both hepatotoxicity and GI bleeding than ibuprofen.

Other NSAIDs are less appropriate, principally for the following reasons:

- Biliary elimination of active forms (indometacin and sulindac) or no biliary elimination information available (naproxen).
- Long half-life (tenoxicam), although this is unlikely to be an issue as long as metabolic capacity remains normal.

Given the rare but potentially hepatotoxic risk with NSAIDs, patients should be instructed to be aware of the symptoms of hepatotoxicity and to report fatigue, malaise, anorexia, nausea and vomiting.

Opioids

Opioids can be used with caution as metabolism is not affected in this patient. Care must be taken to avoid constipation.

- Most opioids have low lipid solubility and are well absorbed orally in cholestasis.
- Most opioids have low protein binding, so alterations in albumin and bilirubin are unlikely to alter free drug levels.
- Cholestasis may reduce the elimination of morphine and possibly codeine, as they undergo some biliary excretion.
- Morphine can reduce biliary secretions and can cause bile duct spasm, which could cause reduced biliary flow, potentially exacerbating this patient's problems. In practice this does not appear to be clinically significant.
- Opioids may worsen this patient's pruritus.

Despite these considerations, in practice standard doses of any opioid can be used in this patient, with monitoring for adverse effects.

Patient 3 – Compensated cirrhosis

Despite cirrhosis, this patient is maintaining good hepatocyte function (normal albumin, mildly raised INR, normal bilirubin) and the metabolic and excretory capacity of the liver should not be significantly reduced. The patient has portal hypertension, so blood flow to the liver will be impaired, which will reduce first-pass metabolism of highly extracted drugs (extraction ratio >0.7). This will result in greater bioavailability of oral doses of these drugs. It is important to note that the patient could rapidly deteriorate into a state of decompensation where liver function would be markedly affected.

Other things to consider are the raised INR and low platelet count (avoid drugs that affect coagulation or cause bleeding), the risk of encephalopathy if the liver function decompensates (caution with any drugs causing sedation, constipation, fluid or electrolyte disturbances) and the risk of hepatorenal syndrome (avoid renally toxic drugs).

Paracetamol

- Paracetamol can safely be administered in normal therapeutic doses in this patient.
- Caution should be used in patients susceptible to hepatic enzyme induction (e.g. chronic alcoholics and patients taking enzyme-inducing drugs). Enzyme induction may theoretically enhance the production of toxic metabolites, but currently there is no clear evidence that these interactions are clinically significant.
- Current evidence suggests that chronic alcoholic patients can be given paracetamol in normal therapeutic doses, as unless they have other risk factors such as malnutrition, their risk of developing severe hepatotoxicity is no greater than that of the general population.
- Caution should be used in patients with reduced ability to eliminate the toxic metabolite due to decreased hepatic stores of glutathione, e.g. malnourished patients.

NSAIDs

NSAIDs should be avoided in this patient, or indeed any patient with cirrhosis, because of their unfavourable side-effect profile:

- Increased risk of bruising/bleeding
- Increased risk of renal dysfunction and hepatorenal syndrome
- Increased risk of gastrointestinal ulceration (especially if taken concomitantly with alcohol)
- Disturbance of electrolytes and fluid balance.

Opioids

Ideally opioids should be avoided in this patient as most are metabolised by the liver and have a high first-pass effect (exceptions include tramadol). There is a risk of increased oral bioavailability in patients with portal hypertension, where blood flow to the liver is reduced, and in patients with cirrhosis where accumulation can occur. The use of any opioid can easily tip a compensated cirrhotic into a state of decompensation because of its side-effect profile. Opioids should only be considered if the patient is in severe pain and unresponsive to other analgesics, but requires careful consideration in all cases. The decision to use them must be reassessed if it is thought that the patient is decompensating. In order to minimise the risk of precipitating decompensation, constipation should be avoided. Where practical, naloxone should also be available to allow for reversal of effects if necessary.

Weak opioids

There is a scarcity of clinical trials regarding the use of codeine and dihydrocodeine in liver impairment; however, they are both metabolised via similar pathways to morphine and dihydromorphine, respectively, and as morphine has been shown to have reduced clearance in cirrhosis the same could be expected of codeine and dihydrocodeine.

Dihydrocodeine

- Preferred weak opioid as its analgesic effect is due primarily to the parent compound rather than an active metabolite formed by the liver.
- Suggested dose: give a single 15 mg dose in adults (0.25 mg/kg in children), monitor for effect and assess appropriate dose and frequency:
  - In practice these types of patients can often tolerate standard doses of 30 mg (adults) and 0.5 mg/kg (children).

Codeine
Should not be considered first line in cirrhotic patients for the following reasons:

- Relies heavily on liver metabolism for conversion to active morphine, so a reduced analgesic effect may be seen.
- Any morphine that is produced will be cleared more slowly.
- Pharmacokinetics of codeine in cirrhotic patients are currently unknown.

Tramadol
Should not be considered first line in cirrhotic patients for the following reasons:

- Tramadol itself acts on the neurotransmitters norepinephrine and sero-tonin, whereas the active intermediate metabolite acts on opioid receptors and has a much higher affinity for these than tramadol.
- If metabolism is reduced the analgesic effect provided by the active metabolite would be expected to decrease.
- The half-life of tramadol and its active metabolite will be increased (owing to reduced clearance) so the overall effect on tramadol activity is not known.
- Tramadol can lower the seizure threshold, which could precipitate seizures in susceptible individuals, e.g. alcoholics.

Strong opioids

These should only be considered in severe pain, preferably after discussion with a liver unit.

Morphine

- Likely to be the strong opioid of choice owing to greatest experience of use.
- Clinical trials have shown that metabolism and clearance of morphine are significantly impaired in patients with cirrhosis, therefore small doses should be used, with reduced frequency of administration.
- It is thought that extrahepatic glucuronidation in the intestine, kidney and brain may increase to compensate for insufficient hepatic metabolism.
- The bioavailability of orally administered morphine is likely to be increased in patients with portal hypertension owing to a reduced first-pass effect, and so lower doses should be used:
  - Suggested starting dose 1.25–2.5 mg in adults and monitor for effect, adjusting dose and frequency accordingly.
- Although the bioavailability of IV/SC/IM dosing is unlikely to be affected in this patient there may still be accumulation of the drug, so a cautious approach should be taken:
  - Start with a dose of 1.25–2.5 mg, monitor for effect, and adjust dose and frequency accordingly.
  - In practice many patients will tolerate a larger dose but will need a reduced frequency to compensate for the decreased clearance.
- Slow-release oral preparations should be avoided as any side effects may be prolonged.

Pethidine

- Should be avoided.
- Has been shown to have approximately a 50% reduction in clearance in patients with cirrhosis.

- Norpethidine, a metabolite of pethidine, which has a longer half-life, may accumulate in cirrhosis, can cause tremor, and also has convulsant properties.

Patient 4 – Decompensated cirrhosis

This patient has decompensated liver disease with significantly impaired synthetic, metabolic and excretory function (low albumin, raised INR, hyperbilirubinaemia, encephalopathy). The reduction in hepatocyte mass and function will significantly reduce the metabolism of low extraction ratio drugs (hepatocyte dependent). The patient also has severe portal hypertension, which will reduce first-pass metabolism, increasing the bioavailability of high extraction ratio drugs. The ascites may alter the absorption and distribution of some drugs. Highly protein-bound drugs may be affected by hypoalbuminaemia and hyperbilirubinaemia, resulting in increased levels of free drug. The cholestasis may impair oral absorption of lipid-soluble drugs and may also reduce biliary excretion.

Other things to consider are the raised INR (avoid drugs that affect coagulation or cause bleeding), encephalopathy (avoid any drugs causing sedation and other CNS side effects, constipation, fluid or electrolyte disturbances) and impaired renal function (adjust doses accordingly and avoid renally toxic drugs).

Paracetamol

The half-life has been shown to be prolonged in some single-dose studies, but no accumulation or hepatotoxicity has been shown after repeated dosing, therefore normal doses and frequency can be used.

Further advice as for Patient 3 with compensated cirrhosis.

NSAIDs

NSAIDs should be avoided in decompensated cirrhotic patients because of the potential for impaired metabolism and increases in the level of unbound drug due to low albumin and high bilirubin, but more importantly NSAIDs should be avoided because of their unfavourable side-effect profile (see details in Patient 3).

Opioids

Ideally opioids should be avoided in this patient, as most are metabolised by the liver so there is a risk of accumulation in hepatic cirrhosis and portal hypertension. This patient is already encephalopathic and any opioid can precipitate or worsen encephalopathy in a patient with decompensated cirrhosis. Opioids should only be considered if the patient is in severe pain and if they are being monitored very closely, ideally as an inpatient. In order to minimise the risk of precipitating or worsening encephalopathy, constipation should be avoided, aiming for two to three regular bowel movements per day. Where practical, naloxone should also be available to allow for reversal of effects if necessary.

Weak opioids

Dihydrocodeine/codeine/tramadol
Advice as for Patient 3, but may require reduced frequency of dosing.

Strong opioids

Should only be considered in very extreme cases, preferably after discussion with a liver unit, and with ICU and respiratory support available.

Morphine
Advice as for Patient 3, but greater care needs to be taken because increased accumulation is likely to occur as the metabolic capacity of the liver is affected in decompensated cirrhosis. Doses at the higher end of the range given are unlikely to be tolerated.

Pethidine
Avoid, as described in Patient 3.

Patient 5 – Acute liver failure

This patient has markedly impaired hepatocyte function and hence reduced metabolic and excretory capacity (raised INR, hyperbilirubinaemia, encephalopathy). Low extraction drugs (hepatocyte dependent) are likely to accumulate and should be used cautiously. The distribution of highly protein-bound drugs may be affected by hyperbilirubinaemia, increasing the unbound fraction. Biliary excretion may be impaired.

Other things to consider are the raised INR (avoid drugs that affect coagulation or cause bleeding), encephalopathy (avoid any drugs causing sedation, constipation, fluid or electrolyte disturbances) and impaired renal function (adjust doses accordingly and avoid renally toxic drugs).

Paracetamol

Because this patient has taken a paracetamol overdose, further administration of paracetamol must be avoided. Glutathione stores will be severely depleted, hence detoxification of the toxic metabolite will be reduced, leading to even greater hepatocyte damage.

Paracetamol could be considered in a patient with acute liver failure caused by something other than a paracetamol overdose. Normal therapeutic doses of paracetamol can be used, but it may be prudent to extend the dosing interval in all patients with acute liver failure because a reduced clearance has been demonstrated in patients with acute viral hepatitis and a prolonged PT.

NSAIDs

NSAIDs should be avoided in any patient with acute liver failure because of their unfavourable side-effect profile.

- Increased risk of bruising/bleeding
- Increased risk of renal dysfunction and hepatorenal syndrome
- Increased risk of gastrointestinal ulceration
- Disturbance of electrolytes and fluid balance.

Opioids

In practice, the metabolism of opioids appears to be well preserved during periods of acute liver dysfunction, but the drugs are likely to accumulate in prolonged disease.

The sedative effects of opioids are dose related, and as this patient has grade III encephalopathy the use of any opioid should be avoided if possible unless the patient is ventilated. Opioids also increase the risk of constipation, leading to worsening encephalopathy. Extreme caution should be exercised with all opioids in patients with renal impairment, as reduced renal excretion can lead to increased and prolonged effects, enhancing respiratory depression, sedation and constipation. Where practical, naloxone should be available to allow for reversal of effects if necessary.

Weak opioids

Dihydrocodeine/codeine/tramadol
As in Patient 3, dihydrocodeine would be the weak opioid of choice with reduced dose and increased dosage interval and daily monitoring of effect.

Strong opioids

These should only be considered in very extreme cases, preferably after discussion with a liver unit, and with ICU and respiratory support available.

Morphine

- Likely to be the strong opioid of choice owing to greatest experience of use.
- Metabolism and clearance of morphine are still likely to be significantly impaired in this patient (note patient also has renal impairment), so small doses should be used with decreased frequency of administration:
  - Start with 1.25–2.5 mg in adults and monitor for effect, adjusting the dose and frequency as necessary.
- Slow-release oral preparations should be avoided as any side effects may be prolonged.

Pethidine
Avoid, as for Patient 3.

References

1. Dollery C (ed) (1999) *Therapeutic Drugs*, 2nd edn. London: Churchill Livingstone.
2. Sweetman S (ed) (2006) *Martindale: The Complete Drug Reference*, 35th edn. London: Pharmaceutical Press.
3. McEvoy GK (ed) (2007) *AHFS Drug Information* 2007. Bethesda, MA: American Society of Health-System Pharmacists.
4. Hutchison TA, Shahan DR, Anderson ML (eds) Drugdex System Internet version Micromedex Inc. Greenwood Village, Colorado (accessed 3 March 2007).
5. Baxter I (ed) (2005) *Stockley's Drug Interactions*, 7th edn. London: Pharmaceutical Press.
6. Brunton LL, Lazo JS, Parker KL, *et al.* (eds) (2005) *Goodman and Gilman's The Pharmacological Basis of Therapeutics*, 11th edn. Maidenhead: McGraw-Hill.

7. Al-O'Baidy SS, McKiernan PJ, Li Wan Po A, *et al*. (1996) Metabolism of paracetamol in children with chronic liver disease. *Eur J Clin Pharmacol* 50: 69–76.

8. Bond R (2004) Reduced toxicity of acetaminophen in children: it's the liver. *Clin Toxicol* 42: 149–152.

9. Vitols S (2003) Paracetamol hepatotoxicity at therapeutic doses. *J Intern Med* 253: 95–98.

10. Watkins P, Kaplowitz N (2006) Aminotransferase elevations in healthy adults receiving 4 grams of acetaminophen daily. *JAMA* 296: 87–93.

11. Bolesta S, Haber SL (2002) Hepatotoxicity associated with chronic acetaminophen administration in patients without risk factors. *Ann Pharmacother* 36: 331–333.

12. Farrell GC (ed) (1994) *Drug-induced Liver Disease*. London: Churchill Livingstone.

13. Makin AJ, Williams R (1997) Acetaminophen-induced hepatotoxicity: predisposing factors and treatments. *Adv Intern Med* 42: 453–483.

14. Prescott LF (2000) Paracetamol, alcohol and the liver. *Br J Clin Pharmacol* 49: 291–301.

15. Whitcomb DC, Block GD (1994) Association of acetaminophen hepatotoxicity with fasting and ethanol use. *JAMA* 272: 1845–1850.

16. Davies DM (ed) (1998) *Textbook of Adverse Drug Reactions*, 5th edn. Oxford: Oxford University Press.

17. Makin AJ, Williams R (2000) Paracetamol hepatotoxicity and alcohol consumption in deliberate and accidental overdose. *QJ Med* 93: 341–349.

18. Thummel KE, Slattery JT, Ro H, *et al*. (2000) Ethanol and production of the hepatotoxic metabolite of acetaminophen in healthy adults. *Clin Pharmacol Ther* 67: 591–599.

19. Kuffner EK, Dart RC, Bogdan GM, *et al*. (2001) Effect of maximal daily doses of acetaminophen on the liver of alcoholic patients. *Arch Intern Med* 161: 2247–2252.

20. Jorup-Ronstrom C, Beerman B, Wahlin-Boll E, *et al*. (1986) Reduction of paracetamol and aspirin metabolism during viral hepatitis. *Clin Pharmacokinet* 11: 250–256.

21. Forrest JAH, Clements JA, Prescott LF (1982) Clinical pharmacokinetics of paracetamol. *Clin Pharmacokinet* 7: 93–107.

22. Leung NW, Critchley JA (1991) Increased oxidative metabolism of paracetamol in patients with hepatocellular carcinoma. *Cancer Lett* 57: 45–48.

23. Personal Communication. Medical Information Department. Roche Products Ltd, Hertfordshire, UK. February 2006.

24. Helleberg L (1981) Clinical pharmacokinetics of indomethacin. *Clin Pharmacokinet* 6: 245–258.

25. Juhl RP, Van Thiel DH, Dittert LW, *et al*. (1983) Ibuprofen and sulindac kinetics in alcoholic liver disease. *Clin Pharmacol Ther* 34: 104–109.

26. Clinoril Summary of Product Characteristics. Merck Sharp & Dohme Limited. Electronic Medicines Compendium. Datapharm Communications Ltd. http: //emc.medicines.org.uk/ (date accessed: March 2007; date of last text revision: November 2003).

27. Aronson JK (ed) (2006) *Meyler's Side Effects of Drugs: The International Encyclopedia of Adverse Drug Reactions and Interactions*, 15th edn. Amsterdam: Elsevier.

28. O'Connor N, Dargan PI, Jones AL (2003) Hepatocellular damage from non-steroidal anti-inflammatory drugs. *QJ Med* 96: 787–791.

29. Zimmerman HJ (ed) (1999) *Hepatotoxicity – the Adverse Effects of Drugs and Other Chemicals on the Liver*, 2nd edn. Baltimore: Lippincott Williams & Wilkins.

30. Rubenstein JH, Laine L (2004) Systematic review: the hepatotoxicity of non-steroidal anti-inflammatory drugs. *Aliment Pharmacol Ther* 20: 373–380.

31. Bush TM, Shlotzhauer TL, Imai K (1991) Nonsteroidal anti-inflammatory drugs: proposed guidelines for monitoring toxicity. *West J Med* 155: 39–42.

32. Garcia-Rodriguez LA, Williams R, Derby LE, *et al.* (1994) Acute liver injury associated with non-steroidal anti-inflammatory drugs and the role of risk factors. *Arch Int Med* 154: 311–316.

33. Davis M (1989) Drugs and abnormal 'liver function tests'. *Adv Drug React Bull* 139: 520–523.

34. Henry D, Lim LL, Garcia-Rodriguez LA, *et al.* (1996) Variability in risk of gastrointestinal complications with individual non-steroidal anti-inflammatory agents – results of a collaborative meta-analysis. *Br Med J* 312: 1563–1566.

35. Brater DC (2002) Anti-inflammatory agents and renal function. *Semin Arthritis Rheum* 32 (Suppl 1): 33–42.

36. Claria J, Kent JD, Lopez-Parra M, *et al.* (2005) Effects of celecoxib and naproxen on renal function in nonazotemic patients with cirrhosis and ascites. *Hepatology* 41: 579–587.

37. Lill JS, O'Sullivan T, Bauer LA, *et al.* (2000) Pharmacokinetics of diclofenac sodium in chronic active hepatitis and alcoholic cirrhosis. *J Clin Pharmacol* 40: 250–257.

38. Voltarol Summary of Product Characteristics, Novartis Pharmaceuticals UK Ltd. Electronic Medicines Compendium. Datapharm Communications Ltd. http://emc.medicines.org.uk/ (date accessed: 6th February 2007, date of last text revision: 8 December 2000).

39. Li G, Treiber G, Maier K, *et al.* (1993) Disposition of ibuprofen in patients with liver cirrhosis. *Clin Pharmacokinet* 25: 154–163.

40. Williams RL, Upton RA, Cello JP, *et al.* (1984) Naproxen disposition in patients with alcoholic cirrhosis. *Eur J Clin Pharmacol* 27: 291–296.

41. Calvo MV, Dominguez A, Macias JG, *et al.* (1980) Naproxen disposition in hepatic and biliary disorders. *Int J Clin Pharmacol Ther Toxicol* 18: 242–246.

42. Nilsen OG (1994) Clinical pharmacokinetics of tenoxicam. *Clin Pharmacokinet* 26: 16–43.

43. Crevoisier CH, Zaugg PY, Heizmann P, *et al.* (1989) Influence of liver cirrhosis upon the pharmacokinetics of tenoxicam. *Int J Clin Pharmacol Res* 9: 327–334.

44. Akriviadis EA, Hatzigavriel M, Kapnias D, *et al.* (1997) Treatment of biliary colic with diclofenac: a randomized, double-blind, placebo-controlled study. *Gastroenterology* 113: 225–231.

45. Koda-Kimble MA, Young LY, Kradjan WA, *et al.* (eds) (2004) *Applied Therapeutics: The Clinical Use of Drugs*, 8th edn. Baltimore: Lippincott, Williams & Wilkins.

46. Personal Communication. Medical Information Department. Napp Pharmaceuticals Ltd. May 2006.

47. Personal Communication. Medical Information Department. Wockhardt UK Ltd. May 2006.

48. Tramadol Summary of Product Characteristics. Pliva. Electronic Medicines Compendium. Datapharm Communications Ltd. http://emc.medicines. org.uk/ (date accessed: 2 March 2007; date of last text revision: June 2003).

49. Grond S, Sablotzki A (2004) Clinical pharmacology of tramadol. *Clin Pharmacokinet* 43: 879–923.

50. Tegeder I, Lotsch J, Geisslinger G (1999) Pharmacokinetics of opioids in liver disease. *Clin Pharmacokinet* 37: 17–40.

51. Poulsen L, Arendt-Nielsen L, Brøsen K, *et al.* (1996) The hypoalgesic effect of tramadol in relation to CYP2D6. *Clin Pharmacol Ther* 60: 636–644.

52. Volles DF, McGory R (1999) Perspectives in pain management – pharmacokinetic considerations. *Crit Care Clin* 15: 55–75.

53. Kluender CN, Klein R, Kohler B (2003) Dramatic increase in bilirubin after ERCP – pethidine as a possible cause of drug-induced hepatitis. *Zeitschr Gastroenterol* 41: 1157–1160.

54. Loughrey MB, Loughrey CM, Johnston S, *et al.* (2003) Fatal hepatic failure following accidental tramadol overdose. *Forensic Sci Int* 134: 232–233.

55. Stricker BHCH (1992) *Drug-induced Hepatic Injury*, 2nd edn. Amsterdam: Elsevier.

56. Anon (1994) Tramadol – a new analgesic. *Drug Ther Bull* 32: 85–87.

57. Pond SM, Tong T, Benowitz NL, *et al.* (1981) Presystemic metabolism of meperidine to normeperidine in normal and cirrhotic subjects. *Clin Pharmacol Ther* 30: 183–188.

58. Patwardhan RV, Johnson RF, Hoyumpa Jr A, *et al.* (1981) Normal metabolism of morphine in cirrhosis. *Gastroenterology* 81: 1006–1011.

59. Hasselstrom J, Eriksson S, Persson A, *et al.* (1990) The metabolism and bioavailability of morphine in patients with severe liver cirrhosis. *Br J Clin Pharmacol* 29: 289–297.

60. Mazoit JX, Sandouk P, Zetlaoui P, *et al.* (1987) Pharmacokinetics of unchanged morphine in normal and cirrhotic subjects. *Anesth Analg* 66: 293–298.

61. Kotb HI, el-Kabsh MY, Emara SE, *et al.* (1997) Pharmacokinetics of controlled release morphine (MST) in patients with liver cirrhosis. *Br J Anaesth* 79: 804–806.

62. Crotty B, Watson KJ, Desmond PV, *et al.* (1989) Hepatic extraction of morphine is impaired in cirrhosis. *Eur J Clin Pharmacol* 36: 501–506.

63. Klotz U, McHorse TS, Wilkinson GR, *et al.* (1974) The effect of cirrhosis on the disposition and elimination of meperidine in man. *Clin Pharmacol Ther* 16: 667–675.

64. McHorse TS, Wilkinson GR, Johnson RF, *et al.* (1975) Effect of acute viral hepatitis in man on the disposition and elimination of meperidine. *Gastroenterology* 68: 775–780.

10

Scenario 2: Choice of antiemetic

Michael Bowe

Summary

Despite the manufacturers of domperidone contraindicating its use in patients with liver disease [1, 2], it is the drug of choice in many liver centres as it has minimal side effects and can be used in all liver patients. In most liver patients the initial starting dose is 10 mg three times a day for adults and 200 µg/kg three times a day for children. However, as domperidone is extensively metabolised by the liver, the initial dose in patients with severe hepatic impairment or cirrhosis should be reduced by 50%, and gradually titrated up to a maximum of 10 mg three times a day, as accumulation of the drug may occur.

The dose of metoclopramide should be reduced by 50% in patients with cirrhosis, as reduced clearance may result in accumulation of the drug. The use of metoclopramide in patients with moderate to severe liver disease may also increase the risk of developing gynae-comastia.

Patients with liver disease may have an increased gastrointestinal transit time [3]. These patients may benefit from taking a pro-kinetic agent, as normalisation of gastrointestinal motility will reduce the time available for the absorption of nitrogenous compounds that may precipitate encephalopathy. The use of pro-kinetic agents has also been shown to reduce intestinal bacterial overgrowth in patients with cirrhosis [4–6].

All $5HT_3$-receptor antagonists are metabolised by the liver, but, with the exception of ondansetron, no dosage adjustments are recommended for the treatment of acute nausea. However, in patients with chronic nausea the dosage of $5HT_3$-receptor antagonist should be reduced to prevent accumulation of the parent drug and any active (or inactive) metabolites.

Table 10.1 Pharmacokinetics of antiemetic drugs in adults

Drug	Bioavailability	T_{max}	Protein binding	Metabolism	% excreted unchanged	Half-life	Active metabolites
Cyclizine		Maximal effects after 1–2 hours		Demethylation to norcyclizine	<1%	20 hours	No
Domperidone	15%	30–60 mins	91–93%	Rapidly and extensively metabolised by hydroxylation and N-dealkylation via CYP3A4, CYP1A2, CYP2E1	10%	7–9 hours	
Granisetron	60% (increased in hepatic impairment)	2 hours	65%	N-demethylation and aromatic ring oxidation followed by conjugation [7]	12%	9 hours (prolonged in hepatic impairment [8])	
Metoclopramide	80%	1–2 hours	30–40%	Low hepatic extraction (<30%). Sulphate conjugation and oxidation reactions via CYP2D6 and CYP3A4 [9]	<25% [9]	5–6 hours (up to 14 hours in cirrhotics [10])	

Table 10.1 Continued

Drug	Bioavailability	T_{max}	Protein binding	Metabolism	% excreted unchanged	Half-life	Active metabolites
Ondansetron	55% (oral) 60% (rectal) (up to 100% in severe hepatic impairment)	1.5 hours (oral) 6 hours (rectal)	70–76%	Indole ring is initially hydroxylated followed by subsequent glucuronide or sulphide conjugation via CYP3A4, CYP2D6, CYP1A2 [7]	<5%	5 hours (oral) 6 hours (rectal) (up to 32 hours in severe hepatic impairment)	Yes – but levels probably too low for clinical activity [7]
Prochlorperazine	0–16%	1.5–5 hours	Unknown but appears to be high	Oxidation and hydroxylation followed by conjugation		7–9 hours	N-desmethyl-prochlor-perazine
Promethazine	25%	2–3 hours (oral) 8 hours (rectal) [11]	76–93%	S-oxidation and N-dealkylation to promethazine sulphoxides and N-demethylpro-methazine [11]		16–19 hours [11]	No

Cyclizine, prochlorperazine and promethazine can be used with caution in patients whose metabolic and synthetic function is unaffected, but must be avoided in encephalopathic patients or in those with cirrhosis who may decompensate.

Unless otherwise stated, all information has been taken from the standard reference sources or the Summary of Product Characteristics [21–27] and refers to adults.

Pharmacokinetics

See Table 10.1 for a summary of pharmacokinetic information.

Absorption

All antiemetics are well absorbed from the gastrointestinal tract, with a C_{max} of 1–2 hours following an oral dose. Domperidone, granisetron, ondansetron, prochlorperazine and promethazine undergo extensive first-pass metabolism, which reduces bioavailability.

Distribution

All antiemetics have low protein binding, except for domperidone (91–93%) and promethazine (93%), and so are unlikely to be affected by alterations in bilirubin or albumin levels, which may result in an increased free fraction in patients with hypoalbuminaemia or hyperbilirubinaemia.

Metabolism

All antiemetics are hepatically metabolised to a lesser or greater degree. Domperidone and prochlorperazine in particular have a very high first-pass effect and are extensively metabolised by the liver.

Elimination

Most antiemetics are excreted via the liver, except metoclopramide, which is primarily removed via the kidneys (80%).

Some relevant adverse effects

Hepatic effects

Hepatic adverse effects secondary to antiemetic therapy are usually asymptomatic. Metoclopramide has been reported as causing cholestasis and the formation of arteriovenous shunts in the liver [12]. The $5HT_3$-receptor antagonists have all been documented as occasionally causing mild increases in liver function tests. Cholestatic jaundice has been reported with cyclizine, prochlorperazine and promethazine, and hepatitis has been reported with cyclizine.

Gastrointestinal effects

Constipation is commonly encountered with cyclizine, owing to its anticholinergic effect. It is also a problem with the $5HT_3$-receptor antagonists as a result of increased gastrointestinal transit time, although the incidence appears to be greater with ondansetron. Dry mouth is seen with cyclizine, prochlorperazine and promethazine. Metoclopramide has been documented as causing diarrhoea.

Neurological effects

Cyclizine commonly causes drowsiness. Other adverse effects reported include blurred vision, restlessness, and auditory and visual hallucinations. Metoclopramide, prochlorperazine and promethazine are all known to cause extrapyramidal effects (most commonly dystonic-type reactions), especially in children and young adults. Drowsiness, restlessness and confusion have also been reported. Domperidone has been reported to cause extrapyramidal effects, but much less frequently than with metoclopramide, as it does not cross the blood–brain barrier. Headache is often seen in patients taking $5HT_3$-receptor antagonists. Visual disturbances and dizziness have also been described in patients taking ondansetron and granisetron. Drowsiness does not appear to be a significant problem with $5HT_3$-receptor antagonists, compared to cyclizine, owing to a lack of effect on H_2 receptors. Extrapyramidal effects have been reported for ondansetron in patients undergoing chemotherapy and for postoperative nausea and vomiting.

Endocrine effects

Metoclopramide, domperidone and prochlorperazine can increase serum prolactin levels, leading to galactorrhoea, irregular periods and gynaecomastia. Raised plasma aldosterone levels have been reported with metoclopramide in both healthy individuals and cirrhotic patients with ascites.

Cardiovascular effects

Arrhythmias have been reported following the use of neuroleptic agents but are not specific to liver disease. However, there may be a greater risk in patients with hepatic impairment owing to accumulation of the drug.

Some relevant drug interactions

Metoclopramide

- Alcohol: Metoclopramide increases the rate of absorption and blood levels of alcohol and increases alcohol-related sedation.
- Paracetamol: Metoclopramide increases the rate of absorption and C_{max} of paracetamol.
- Morphine: Metoclopramide increases the rate of absorption, rate of onset and sedative effects of morphine.
- Ciclosporin: Metoclopramide increases the rate of absorption and serum levels of ciclosporin – monitor ciclosporin levels closely.

Domperidone

Nil of note.

Granisetron

Nil of note.

Cyclizine

- Alcohol: Increased sedative effect.

Prochlorperazine

- Alcohol: Increased sedative effect.

- Desferrioxamine: Simultaneous administration should be avoided as transient metabolic encephalopathy, characterised by loss of consciousness for 48–72 hours, has been reported.

Promethazine

- Alcohol: Increased sedative effect.
- Opioids: Promethazine reduces the required analgesic and anaesthetic doses of several opioids. Sedation is also increased.

Clinical studies

Metoclopramide

Metoclopramide is classified as having a low hepatic extraction (<30%) and a low protein-binding affinity (<90%). This means that the absolute bioavailability of metoclopramide is not grossly affected in the cirrhotic patient but that its clearance may be reduced owing to impaired hepatic metabolism [3]. Despite metoclopramide being cleared renally, several small studies have compared its pharmacokinetics in both healthy volunteers and in patients with severe cirrhosis. The results show that the rate of clearance is reduced by 50% in the cirrhotic group, suggesting impaired renal clearance secondary to cirrhosis, even in patients with apparently normal creatinine. As a result, it is recommended that the dose of metoclopramide is reduced by 50% in patients with severe cirrhosis, as accumulation of the drug may occur [10, 13, 14]. (The dose should also be reduced according to the patient's renal function.)

Metoclopramide has been shown to significantly reduce spironolactone-induced diuresis in cirrhotic patients with ascites. When administered to patients with secondary hyperaldosteronism, metoclopramide significantly reduced urinary sodium excretion, with a corresponding increase in urinary potassium excretion and a significant increase in plasma aldosterone. This effect was not seen with domperidone. From this study it is recommended that metoclopramide is avoided during diuretic therapy in cirrhotic patients with ascites [15].

Domperidone

No clinical studies have been performed using domperidone in patients with liver disease.

Ondansetron

As the primary route of elimination is hepatic metabolism, the clearance of ondansetron is affected by liver disease. A study in 12 patients with varying degrees of hepatic insufficiency (based on the Pugh score) showed a reduced first-pass metabolic effect compared with matched controls. Patients with mild (Pugh scores 6 and 7) to moderate (Pugh scores 8 and 9) hepatic impairment demonstrated a twofold reduction in clearance and a twofold increase in mean half-life. In severe hepatic impairment (Pugh score >9) clearance was reduced two- to threefold and volume of distribution was increased, resulting in a mean half-life of 20 hours (5.7 hours in normal controls). Following oral administration changes in mean absolute bioavailability – approaching 100% compared to 66% in normal controls – are also seen in severe hepatic impairment. This is believed to be due to an impaired metabolic clearance, resulting in a significantly reduced first-pass effect [16]. As a result of this study, the following dosing information is to be found on the Summary of Product Characteristics for ondansetron: GlaxoSmithKline state that the 'clearance of Zofran [ondansetron] is significantly reduced and the serum half-life significantly prolonged in patients with moderate or severe impairment of hepatic function. In such patients a total daily dose of 8 mg should not be exceeded' [17].

It is known that $5HT_3$ receptors on the dermal sensory nerve endings are involved in the sensation of itch. The antipruritic effect of ondansetron has been investigated, but the results have been inconclusive. One small double-blind, placebo-controlled trial ($n = 19$), in which patients had taken ondansetron 8 mg twice daily for a five-day period, found no benefit over placebo [18]. Another study randomised patients to ondansetron 8 mg three times a day or placebo for one week and demonstrated a small, but significant, improvement in itch scores with the active therapy (although ondansetron was not preferred over placebo by the patients) [19].

Ondansetron has also been investigated for the treatment of fatigue associated with primary biliary cirrhosis but results have been disappointing. A randomised, controlled crossover trial ($n = 54$) examined the effect of ondansetron 4 mg three times a day versus placebo for a four-week period, before being crossed over for a further four-week period. The study concluded that the use of ondansetron did not offer a clinically significant reduction in fatigue compared to placebo [20]. However, the results of the study may have been affected as patients were effectively unblinded during the second phase of the study as a result of side effects to ondansetron (constipation 63% vs 13%).

Granisetron

One small study examined the pharmacokinetics and efficacy of granisetron in patients with or without metastatic liver disease. This open-labelled, single intravenous dose, comparative study was designed to show any pharmacokinetic changes in patients with hepatic dysfunction. The hepatically impaired group showed a 50% reduction in total clearance compared to those patients with normal liver function. The authors concluded that '...although hepatically impaired patients had higher mean area under the curve values, the observed values were in a range that was similar to ranges observed in patients and healthy volunteers who have received higher doses of granisetron in other studies. Therefore, it is unlikely that the observed differences have any clinical implications' [8]. As this was a single-dose study it makes it difficult to extrapolate the data to repeated dosing. The patients involved had metastatic liver disease, but none was reported to be cirrhotic. As granisetron has a high first-pass metabolism, it would seem prudent to reduce the dose in the cirrhotic patient.

Cyclizine, prochlorperazine and promethazine

There is a paucity of data examining the use of these agents in patients with hepatic impairment. Although there is no information available to recommend any necessary dosage adjustments in hepatic impairment, their use should be avoided in moderate to severe liver disease, owing to their sedative adverse effects.

CASE STUDIES

See Appendix 1 for full patient details.

Patient 1 – Mild hepatitis without cirrhosis

The synthetic and metabolic capacity of this patient's liver is unlikely to be affected by the isolated rise in ALT. Drug handling is unlikely to be altered. It is important to ensure that the patient has no signs of cirrhosis, as many diseases that present with this clinical picture can become cirrhotic despite near normal laboratory tests.

- Metoclopramide, domperidone or 5HT$_3$-receptor antagonists could be used in this patient, taking into account the usual considerations when using these drugs.
- Cyclizine, prochlorperazine or promethazine could be used as the patient is not at risk of encephalopathy.
- LFTs should be monitored with drugs known to cause rises in LFTs or hepatotoxicity, as well as for deterioration in liver function.
- Any change in the patient's clinical condition should prompt a review of the prescription.

Patient 2 – Cholestasis

The synthetic and metabolic capacity of this patient's liver is unlikely to be affected by cholestasis. However, consideration needs to be given to protein binding (patient has hyperbilirubinaemia); excretion of the drug or metabolites in bile (patient has cholestasis); and lipophilicity of the drug (some lipophilic drugs require bile salts for absorption and these would be reduced in cholestasis).

- Metoclopramide, domperidone, ondansetron and granisetron are not highly protein bound, so they are unlikely to be affected by changes in albumin and bilirubin.
- The biliary excretion of metoclopramide is approximately 5%, so elimination is unlikely to be affected (main route of elimination is renal).
- Ondansetron may be the drug of choice in this patient as they are also suffering itch. As there is no change in the patient's metabolic function, a dose of 4–8 mg (50–100 µg/kg in children) two or three times daily could be used. Rifampicin may reduce the antiemetic effect.
- Granisetron could be used.
- Cyclizine, prochlorperazine or promethazine could be used as the patient is not at risk of encephalopathy.
- LFTs should be monitored with drugs known to cause rises in LFTs or hepatotoxicity, as well as for deterioration in liver function.
- Any change in the patient's clinical condition should prompt a review of the prescription.

Patient 3 – Compensated cirrhosis

Despite cirrhosis, this patient is maintaining good hepatocyte function (normal albumin and bilirubin, mildly raised INR) and the metabolic and excretory capacity of the liver should not be significantly reduced. The patient has portal hypertension, so blood flow to the liver will be impaired, which will reduce first-pass metabolism of highly extracted drugs (extraction ratio >0.7). This will result in greater bioavailability of oral doses of these drugs. It is important to note that the patient could rapidly deteriorate into a state of decompensation where liver function would be markedly affected.

Other things to consider are the raised INR and low platelet count (avoid drugs that affect coagulation or cause bleeding), the risk of encephalopathy if the liver function decompensates (caution with any drugs causing sedation, constipation, fluid or electrolyte disturbances) and the risk of hepatorenal syndrome (avoid renally toxic drugs).

- Domperidone may be the antiemetic of choice in this patient. Despite being extensively metabolised by the liver it has few adverse effects and does not cross the blood–brain barrier.
- Metoclopramide could be used in an older patient, but as this patient is only 14 years old it should be avoided, where possible, because of the increased incidence of extrapyramidal effects in children, young adults and females. In an older patient, an initial dose of 10 mg three times a day could be used and then titrated against response and adverse effects.
- Cyclizine, prochlorperazine or promethazine could be used with caution but the sedative effects may mask the development of encephalopathy.
- Ondansetron could be used, but the dose should be reduced to 8 mg daily in divided doses.
- Granisetron could be used.

Patient 4 – Decompensated cirrhosis

This patient has decompensated liver disease with significantly impaired synthetic, metabolic and excretory function (low albumin, raised INR, hyperbilirubinaemia, encephalopathy). The reduction in hepatocyte mass and function will significantly reduce the metabolism of low extraction ratio drugs (hepatocyte dependent). The patient also has severe portal hypertension, which will reduce first-pass metabolism, thereby increasing the bioavailability of high extraction ratio drugs. The ascites and cholestasis may affect the absorption of some drugs and ascites may alter the distribution of hydrophilic drugs. Highly protein-bound drugs may be affected by hypoalbuminaemia and hyperbilirubin-aemia, resulting in increased levels of free drug. Cholestasis may reduce the biliary excretion of some drugs.

Other things to consider are the raised INR (avoid drugs that affect coagulation or cause bleeding), encephalopathy (avoid any drugs causing sedation and other CNS side effects, constipation, fluid or electrolyte disturbances) and impaired renal function (adjust doses accordingly and avoid renally toxic drugs).

- Domperidone may be the antiemetic of choice in this patient. Despite being extensively metabolised by the liver it has few adverse effects and does not cross the blood–brain barrier. The bioavailability is likely to be increased as first-pass metabolism will be reduced because of portal hypertension. There may also be accumulation of domperidone owing to reduced metabolic capacity. Consequently the dose should be reduced to 50% and titrated up to 10 mg three times a day if necessary.
- Ondansetron could be used, but the dose should be reduced to 8 mg daily in divided doses, as this patient has severe hepatic impairment (Child–Pugh C). Ondansetron should be used with caution as it can cause constipation, which may worsen encephalopathy. A laxative should be co-prescribed if necessary.
- Granisetron could be used, starting at 1 mg daily and increasing where necessary.
- Metoclopramide should be avoided where possible, as it may cause cerebral irritation. If metoclopramide were to be used the dose should be reduced to 50% of normal, because of reduced hepatic clearance and concomitantly reduced renal clearance. The dose may also require further reduction according to renal function. As this patient is currently taking spironolactone, metoclopramide should be avoided as it may reduce the diuretic effect.
- Cyclizine, prochlorperazine and promethazine should be avoided as they may mask the development of encephalopathy.

Patient 5 – Acute liver failure

This patient has markedly impaired hepatocyte function and consequently reduced metabolic and excretory capacity (raised INR, hyperbilirubinaemia, encephalopathy). Low extraction drugs (hepatocyte dependent) are likely to accumulate and should be used cautiously. The distribution of highly protein-bound drugs may be affected by hyperbilirubinaemia, increasing the unbound fraction. Biliary excretion may be impaired.

Other things to consider are the raised INR (avoid drugs that affect coagulation or cause bleeding), encephalopathy (avoid any drugs causing sedation, constipation, fluid or electrolyte disturbances) and impaired renal function (adjust doses accordingly and avoid renally toxic drugs).

- As the patient is grade III encephalopathic and is likely to be ventilated, there is probably no need for any antiemetic therapy.
- In patients with grade I or II encephalopathy the use of antiemetics should be avoided where possible, as the patient may have fluctuating levels of consciousness and cerebral function.

- Domperidone may be the antiemetic of choice, but as the patient has very little metabolic and synthetic liver function, owing to massive hepato-cellular necrosis secondary to the hepatotoxic effects of the paracetamol overdose, accumulation of the domperidone may occur. However, it may be of benefit as a pro-kinetic agent.
- Metoclopramide is best avoided, as there is an increased risk of it causing cerebral irritation.
- Ondansetron could be used, but the dose should be reduced to 4 mg once a day as this patient has very little metabolic and synthetic liver function.

In the conscious patient with acute liver failure antiemetics should be avoided where possible, but ondansetron 8 mg (or less) daily may be used.

References

1. Winthrop Pharmaceuticals UK Ltd (2004) Motilium tablets 10 mg. Summary of Product Characteristics.
2. Wockhardt UK Ltd (2005) Domperidone tablets 10 mg. Summary of Product Characteristics.
3. Delcò F, Tchambaz L, Schlienger R *et al.* (2005) Dose adjustment in patients with liver disease. *Drug Safety* 28: 529–545.
4. Xiang-Sheng F, Feng J (2006) Cisapride decreasing orocecal transit time in patients with non-alcoholic steatohepatitis. *Hepatobiliary Pancreat Dis Int* 5: 534–537.
5. Pardo A, Bartoli R, Lorenzo-Zuniga V, *et al.* (2000) Effect of cisapride on intestinal bacterial overgrowth and bacterial translocation in cirrhosis. *Hepatology* 31: 858–863.
6. Madrid AM, Hurtado C, Venegas M, *et al.* (2001) Long-term treatment with cisapride and antibiotics in liver cirrhosis: effect on small intestine motility, bacterial overgrowth, and liver function. *Am J Gastroenterol* 96: 1251–1255.
7. Kok-Yuen H, Tong JG (2005) Pharmacology, pharmacogenetics, and clinical efficacy of 5-hydroxytrytamine type 3 receptor antagonists for postoperative nausea and vomiting. *Curr Opin Anaesthesiol* 19: 606–611.
8. Palmer R (1994) Efficacy and safety of granisetron (Kytril) in two special populations: Children and adults with impaired hepatic function. *Semin Oncol* 21(Suppl 5): 22–25.
9. Desta Z, Wu GM, Morocho AM, *et al.* (2002) The gastroprokinetic and antiemetic drug metoclopramide is a substrate and inhibitor of cytochrome P450 2D6. *Drug Metab Dispos* 30: 336–343.
10. Bernardi M, Tamè MR, Albani F, *et al.* (1991) Pharmacokinetics of metoclopramide after single oral dose administration in cirrhosis. *Eur J Gastroenterol Hepatol* 3: 519–522.
11. Strenkoski-Nix LC, Ermer J, DeCleene S, *et al.* (2000) Pharmacokinetics of promethazine hydrochloride after administration of rectal suppositories and oral syrup to healthy subjects. *Am J Health-Syst Pharm* 57: 1499–1505.

12. Feurle GE (1990) Arteriovenous shunting and cholestasis in hepatic hemangiomatosis associated with metoclopramide. *Gastroenterology* 99: 258–262.

13. Magueur E, Horgege H, Attali P, *et al.* (1991) Pharmacokinetics of metoclopramide in patients with liver cirrhosis. *Br J Clin Pharmacol* 31: 185–187.

14. Albani F, Tamè MR, De Palma R, *et al.* (1991) Kinetics of intravenous metoclopramide in patients with hepatic cirrhosis. *Eur J Clin Pharmacol* 40: 423–425.

15. D'Arienzo A, Ambrogio G, Di Siervi P, *et al.* (1985) A randomised comparison of metoclopramide and domperidone on plasma aldosterone concentration and on spironolactone-induced diuresis in ascitic cirrhotic patients. *Hepatology* 5: 854–857.

16. Figg WD, Dukes GE, Pritchard JF, *et al.* (1996) Pharmacokinetics of ondansetron in patients with hepatic insufficiency. *J Clin Pharmacol* 36: 206–215.

17. GlaxoSmithKline UK (2006) Zofran tablets. Summary of Product Characteristics.

18. O'Donohue JW, Pereira SP, Ashdown AC, *et al.* (2005) A controlled trial of ondansetron in the pruritus of cholestasis. *Aliment Pharmacol Ther* 21: 1041–1045.

19. Muller C, Pongratz S, Pidlich J, *et al.* (1998) Treatment of pruritus in chronic liver disease with the 5-hydroxytryptamine receptor type 3 antagonist ondansetron: A randomized, placebo-controlled, double-blind cross-over trial. *Eur J Gastroenterol Hepatol* 10: 865–870.

20. Theal JJ, Toosi MN, Girlan L, *et al.* (2005) A randomized, controlled crossover trial of ondansetron in patients with primary biliary cirrhosis and fatigue. *Hepatology* 41: 1305–1312.

21. Dollery C (ed) (1999) *Therapeutic Drugs,* 2nd edn. London: Churchill Livingstone.

22. Sweetman S (ed) (2005) *Martindale: The Complete Drug Reference,* 34th edn. London: Pharmaceutical Press.

23. McEvoy GK (ed) (2006) *AHFS Drug Information.* Bethesda, MA: American Society of Health-System Pharmacists.

24. Hutchison TA, Shahan DR, Anderson ML (eds) (2007) *Drugdex System* Internet version Micromedex Inc. Greenwood Village, Colorado (accessed 9 May 2007).

25. Baxter I (ed) (2005) *Stockley's Drug Interactions,* 7th edn. London: Pharmaceutical Press.

26. Mehta DK (ed) (2007) *British National Formulary.* No. 53. London: British Medical Association and Royal Pharmaceutical Society.

27. Aronson JK (ed) (2006) *Meyler's Side Effects of Drugs: The International Encyclopedia of Adverse Drug Reactions and Interactions,* 15th edn. Amsterdam: Elsevier.

11

Scenario 3: Choice of anti-hyperlipidaemic agent

Fionnuala Kennedy

Summary

When choosing an anti-hyperlipidaemic drug for a patient, it is important to consider that most of these drugs are primarily metabolised by the liver. The standard patient counselling is recommended and special attention should be paid to:

- Myalgia, myopathy and rhabdomyolysis
- Signs of bleeding, such as bruising, bleeding gums and the symptoms of anaemia.

  In general:

- Lipid-lowering therapy may not be 'urgent' and consideration should be given to holding therapy until any acute liver episode has passed and the patient is compensated.
- Consider that a patient might decompensate: a drug which is unlikely to accumulate in this situation is preferable.
- In cirrhosis, preference should be given to drugs that are not primarily metabolised and/or eliminated through the liver.
- In cirrhosis the first-pass effect is significantly reduced, and this may lead to greatly elevated concentrations of drug reaching the systemic circulation. Most statins and fibrates have a high first-pass extraction.
- Initial doses should be at the lower end of the scale and should be increased cautiously.
- Consider potential drug interactions, some of which may be serious or even fatal, particularly in relation to the statins.
- Drugs which are highly protein bound (most statins, fibrates and ezetimibe) should be used with caution in hypoalbuminaemia and hyperbilirubinaemia.
- Drugs that affect coagulation (e.g. niacin, fibrates) should be avoided or used with caution in coagulopathy or in patients who have previously decompensated or who have varices/portal hypertension. They may also

exacerbate the anticoagulant effect of other drugs that alter INR, PT, or cause thrombocytopenia or anaemia.

- Niacin and acipimox should be avoided in patients with gastritis or varices.
- In hepatorenal syndrome (HRS), which is an acute episode, the clearance of renally excreted drugs and metabolites (pravastatin, simvastatin, rosuvastatin, acipimox, fibrates) may be reduced. During an episode of HRS, anti-hyperlipidaemic medication should be withheld.

Before treating a patient's hyperlipidaemia with drugs, other options such as diet and exercise should be considered.

Statins

The Summary of Product Characteristics (SPC) for each product states that all statins are contraindicated in *active* liver disease and in patients with persistent unexplained elevations of liver enzymes exceeding three times the upper limit of normal (ULN) [1, 2]. This is due to their extensive liver metabolism, their ability to cause raised transaminases and the risk of myopathy or rhabdomyolysis in the presence of reduced synthetic function, or to a drug interaction that reduces their metabolism.

Nonetheless, statins can probably be used safely in liver disease where there is no synthetic dysfunction, and even where there is a degree of liver dysfunction, provided the *appropriate* agent is used at an *appropriate* dose. *This is in direct contradiction to the SPC for each product and must be borne in mind by clinicians when considering statin therapy.* Starting doses should be low (e.g. pravastatin 10 mg or simvastatin 10 mg at night) and the dose must be increased cautiously. Simvastatin may be used in patients with no synthetic dysfunction, although if cirrhosis and synthetic dysfunction subsequently develop, pravastatin would be a more suitable choice.

Patients must be monitored carefully for signs of myopathy and hepatotoxicity. Elevations of transaminases as a possible pharmacodynamic effect of lipid-lowering therapy should be considered. Liver function tests (LFTs) should be monitored to identify possible hepatotoxicity. Statins should be withheld or changed if elevations in transaminases are persistently more than three times ULN or are accompanied by other signs of liver disease that might be iatrogenic. In addition, the patient must be adequately monitored in order to identify:

- An episode of decompensation which might result in reduced clearance of the drug.

- Reduced renal clearance of pravastatin and rosuvastatin in the presence of HRS; during an episode of HRS, anti-hyperlipidaemic medication should be withheld.
- Reduced excretion through bile in obstructive cholestasis (use a statin that is partially cleared in the urine).

Based on their pharmacokinetic profile alone, the safest statins in chronic compensated liver disease and a history of decompensation are probably pravastatin and rosuvastatin. However, clinical experience with rosuvastatin in liver disease is lacking, and so it cannot be recommended. In addition, the true rate of post-marketing adverse drug reactions is not yet clear. Pravastatin is therefore the drug of choice in these patients, where treatment is deemed necessary. It should, however, be avoided in acute episodes until liver function or transaminases stabilise/return to normal.

In 2006 the National Lipid Association's Statin Safety Assessment Task Force concluded that chronic liver disease and compensated liver disease are not contraindications to the use of statins, but that they are contraindicated in decompensated disease or liver failure [2, 3]; see Hepatic Adverse Effects.

Bile acid sequestrants

Bile acid sequestrants should be used with caution in constipation and avoided in complete biliary obstruction or in patients at risk of decompensation. Vitamin K absorption may be reduced and the INR/PT should be monitored. Oral vitamin K supplementation should not be administered at the same time of day. There should be an adequate interval between the administration of bile acid sequestrants and other drugs.

Fibrates

Fibrate absorption may be reduced in the presence of cholestasis. Metabolism will be reduced in liver dysfunction. Renal failure increases the risk of myopathy with fibrate use. During an episode of HRS, anti-hyperlipidaemic medication should be withheld.

Fibrates should be avoided in gallbladder disease or any form of obstructive jaundice because of the risk of stone formation. The extended therapeutic effect of gemfibrozil, which is due to enterohepatic recycling, may be reduced in obstructive jaundice. Fibrates may have an adverse effect on coagulation: if used, the INR/PT should be monitored and the dose of anticoagulant altered accordingly. They are highly protein bound.

Selective cholesterol absorption inhibitors

Ezetimibe is usually used in combination with simvastatin. Patients should be monitored for signs of myopathy. Monitor transaminases. The extended therapeutic effect due to enterohepatic recycling may be reduced in obstructive jaundice.

Inhibitors of fasting-induced lipolysis

Niacin and acipimox should be relatively safe to use in the absence of varices, gastritis, coagulopathy, thrombocytopenia or a history of decompensation. Both can cause pruritus, which is common in cholestatic liver disease. The extended release formulation of niacin (Niaspan® Prolonged Release) may cause hepatitis and LFTs should be monitored.

Background

Hyperlipidaemia may occur independently of, or as a result of, liver disease. When it occurs secondary to liver disease, it tends to manifest as hypercholesterolaemia [4–7]. There are three liver disorders in which it commonly occurs:

- Primary biliary cirrhosis (PBC)
- Primary sclerosing cholangitis (PSC)
- Non-alcoholic steatohepatitis (NASH) or non-alcoholic fatty liver disease (NAFLD).

It is less likely in other forms of liver disease, such as acute hepatitis and cirrhosis. Cirrhosis may actually protect against atherosclerosis [5, 8, 9]. The reasons for this are not clear. Secondary hypercholesterolaemia frequently occurs in cholestatic conditions, but usually does not require treatment [10]. Other risk factors for hyperlipidaemia and cardiovascular disease should be assessed, as their presence may independently indicate a need for medical intervention [9]. In PBC, patients with severe, chronic disease do not appear to have an increased cardiovascular risk as a result of their hypercholesterolaemia: this may be due to the presence of cirrhosis. In contrast, in less severe PBC patients with moderate hypercholesterolaemia there appears to be an increased cardiovascular risk, which may be due to the absence of the protective effect of cirrhosis [7].

Patients with NASH/NAFLD frequently have elevated serum triglycerides. In two small studies treatment has been shown to improve serum cholesterol and reduce transaminases, although the value of such treatment needs to be further investigated [11, 12].

Hyperlipidaemia is common after transplantation, with an increased risk of ischaemic heart disease and cardiovascular complications. These patients are on lifelong immunosuppressive drugs. Hyperlipidaemia is associated with the long-term use of ciclosporin, to a lesser extent tacrolimus, high-dose steroids and, in particular, sirolimus, which commonly causes elevated triglycerides [1]. It is more prevalent in renal and cardiac transplant recipients [13–15]. In one liver transplant study, serum cholesterol >5 mmol/L was found in 44% of recipients. Compared to age- and sex-matched controls, the relative risk for ischaemic cardiac events was 3.07 and for cardiovascular deaths 2.56 [16]. The combination of diabetes mellitus and known coronary artery disease prior to transplant may reduce five-year survival by up to 40% after liver transplantation. Risk factors in these patients need to be treated aggressively. In the absence of recurrent liver disease, treatment is as for the general population. However, some liver transplant recipients go on to develop recurrent liver disease. The time-scale varies greatly and may be as little as six months for hepatitis C. In patients transplanted for conditions with an autoimmune component (e.g. autoimmune hepatitis, PSC, PBC), the disease may recur after five to 20 years. As a result, the possibility of liver disease needs to be taken into consideration when prescribing anti-hyperlipidaemic therapy in liver transplant recipients.

There are five classes of medication used to treat hyperlipidaemia:

- Statins (HMG-CoA-reductase inhibitors)
- Bile acid sequestrants
- Fibrates
- Selective cholesterol absorption inhibitor
- Inhibitors of fasting-induced lipolysis.

Pharmacokinetics

See Table 11.1 for a summary of pharmacokinetic information relating to drugs used in hyperlipidaemia [1, 17–19].

Table 11.1 Pharmacokinetics of anti-hyperlipidaemic agents in adults

	Total absorption (%)	Activity	First-pass effects (%)	Systemic bioavailability (%)
Atorvastatin	30	Active, active metabolites	>70	12–14
Fluvastatin	98	Active	70	19–29
Pravastatin	34	Active, minor active metabolites	50	17–18
Rosuvastatin	50	Active, minor active metabolites	63	20
Simvastatin (prodrug)	60–80 Extensive	Prodrug, active metabolites, converted mainly in liver	78–87, Extensive	5
Colestyramine	0	N/A	N/A	N/A
Colestipol	0	N/A	N/A	N/A
Bezafibrate	100	Active	None	100
Ciprofibrate	>99, rapid	Suggested that it may be converted to an active ester, primarily in liver	Minimal	High

Table 11.1 Continued

	Total absorption (%)	Activity	First-pass effects (%)	Systemic bioavailability (%)
Fenofibrate	30–50 (fasting) 60–90 (food)	Prodrug which is rapidly and completely hydrolyzed by plasma and tissue esterases to fenofibric acid	To active fenofibric acid (see activity)	High (fenofibric acid)
Gemfibrozil	100	Active, minor active metabolite	None	Significant enterohepatic recirculation
Ezetimibe	Rapid	Active glucuronide metabolite	Extensively glucuronidated to active form in intestine wall and liver	Significant enterohepatic recirculation with transformation to and reabsorption of ezetimibe prolongs half-life
Acipimox	Rapid and complete > 90	Active	Negligible	High
Niacin (nicotinic acid)	> 90, rapid	Active	Saturable system	Depends on level of saturation of first pass metabolism

N/A = not applicable.

(continued)

Table 11.1 Continued

	Lipophilicity	Protein binding (%)	Metabolism	Renal excretion (%)	Faecal excretion (%)
Atorvastatin	Lipophilic	80–90	3A4	< 5	90
Fluvastatin	Lipophilic	99	2C9 (major) 2D6, 3A4 (both minor)	5	95
Pravastatin	Hydrophilic	50	Minor, some sulphation	20	71
Rosuvastatin	Hydrophilic	88	Minor: 10% (2C9 and to a lesser extent 2C19)	10	90, mostly unchanged
Simvastatin	Lipophilic	94–98	3A4 Glucuronidation	13	58–60
Colestyramine	N/A	N/A	N/A	N/A	100
Colestipol	N/A	N/A	N/A	N/A	100
Bezafibrate	Lipophilic	94–96	Glucuronides and polar metabolites	94–95, half of which is unchanged drug	3
Ciprofibrate	Hydrophobic	95	Extensive glucuronidation	Extensive 7% unchanged drug)	3

Table 11.1 Continued

	Lipophilicity	Protein binding (%)	Metabolism	Renal excretion (%)	Faecal excretion (%)
Fenofibrate	Hydrophobic	99	Glucuronidation carbonyl reduction	60–88	25
Gemfibrozil	>1/1000 water	97	Glucuronidation hydroxylation oxidation in liver	70, mainly as conjugates and metabolites, 6% unchanged drug	6% faeces
Ezetimibe	Hydrophobic	99.7 (ezetimibe) and 88–92 (glucuronide)	Glucuronide cleared slowly from plasma	11	78
Acipimox	Relatively hydrophilic	Negligible	Little	90 unchanged	5
Niacin (nicotinic acid)	Relatively hydrophilic	15–30	Saturable liver, extensive	60–76 total dose (12% dose as unchanged drug)	

N/A = not applicable.

Absorption and first-pass effect

General considerations

The absorption of highly lipophilic drugs (atorvastatin, simvastatin, ezetimibe, fibrates) may be reduced in cholestasis if they require bile salts for their absorption.

The first-pass effect may be reduced in cirrhosis and portal hypertension owing to reduced blood flow through the liver. Additionally, in cirrhosis and acute hepatitis the number of functional hepatocytes may be reduced. Drugs with a high first-pass extraction ratio and a narrow therapeutic window, such as the statins, are more likely to be toxic in patients with liver dysfunction [20]. In liver disease, an increase in the percentage of drug reaching the systemic circulation is an important factor in statin toxicity.

Statins (HMG-CoA-reductase inhibitors)

The statins, except for fluvastatin, are poorly absorbed from the gastro-intestinal tract [19].They are generally hepatoselective. More lipophilic statins diffuse passively into hepatocytes, and more hydrophilic statins are actively taken up by an organic anion transport protein (OATP) [21]. They are more hepatoselective than the lipophilic statins.

Most undergo a high extraction on first pass through the liver and systemic bioavailability is low (5–29%) in patients with normal liver function [1, 17, 19]. Simvastatin is a lactone prodrug that requires conversion by esterases to the active open acid form [19]. In humans this is thought to take place in the liver.

Atorvastatin is absorbed well but is subject to extensive first-pass metabolism in the gut wall and the liver, converting it to active metabolites that are responsible for 70% of its clinical activity [19, 22].

Bile acid sequestrants

Not absorbed, as their therapeutic effect is exerted in the gut.

Fibrates

Fibrates, except for immediate-release fenofibrate, are generally well absorbed [1, 19]. They do not undergo first-pass extraction.

Ezetimibe

Ezetimibe is well absorbed and rapidly glucuronidated [1]. The glucuronide undergoes extensive enterohepatic recycling, resulting in multiple peaks. It is more active than the parent drug [1].

Inhibitors of fasting-induced lipolysis

Acipimox and niacin are absorbed rapidly and completely [1, 19].

Distribution

Statins (HMG-CoA-reductase inhibitors)

Most statins are highly plasma protein bound and highly lipophilic. The exceptions are pravastatin and rosuvastatin, but it is not known whether they distribute into ascitic fluid [19, 21]. The statins, except possibly rosuvastatin and fluvastatin, are substrates for P-glycoprotein, a pump which is responsible for the excretion of drugs back into the gut, from where they may be reabsorbed or excreted in the faeces [23, 24].

Fibrates

The fibrates are all highly protein bound. Gemfibrozil undergoes enterohepatic recycling [1, 19].

Ezetimibe

Ezetimibe is highly lipid soluble. Both the parent drug and the active glucuronide are highly plasma protein bound [1].

Inhibitors of fasting-induced lipolysis

Both acipimox and niacin are poorly protein bound and quite hydrophilic [19]. It is not known whether they distribute into ascitic fluid.

Metabolism

Statins (HMG-CoA-reductase inhibitors)

Glucuronide formation appears to be a common route of clearance for the hydroxyl-acid form of statins, converting them to an inactive δ-lactone derivative [17, 25].

Although atorvastatin is administered as an active form, 70% of its activity is due to hydroxylated CYP3A4 metabolites [19]. Atorvastatin is metabolised in the gut wall and the liver [22].

The hydrophilic statins (pravastatin, rosuvastatin) are only partly metabolised by the liver [1, 17, 19]. Pravastatin is also metabolised in the stomach [26]. The pharmacokinetics of pravastatin have been shown to change in liver disease, despite its dual route (renal and hepatic) of elimination [27]. Nonetheless, it has been used in liver disease and has been suggested as the statin of choice [26]. Liver metabolism is of minor importance in the clearance of rosuvastatin and its pharmacokinetics are not altered by mild to moderate liver impairment. However, the area under the curve (AUC) is increased in severe liver impairment [1]. Clinical experience with rosuvastatin in liver disease is lacking, and it therefore cannot be recommended.

Hepatic disease has been shown to reduce the clearance of atorvastatin, pravastatin, fluvastatin and simvastatin, and renal disease reduces the clearance of simvastatin [28], reflecting their various pathways of metabolism and subsequent elimination. The AUC of atorvastatin is increased 11-fold in Child–Pugh class B chronic alcoholic liver disease. Exposure to pravastatin is increased by 50% in alcoholic cirrhosis [1]. Simvastatin is a lactone prodrug that requires conversion by esterases to the active open acid form, simvastatin acid [19]. This is thought to take place in the liver in humans and may be reduced in the presence of reduced metabolic function or cirrhosis, resulting in greatly increased exposure to the parent prodrug. However, this must be set against a reduced first-pass effect causing decreased levels of the active acid.

Fibrates

In general, the fibrates are glucuronidated by hepatic enzymes and may accumulate in liver dysfunction [1, 19].

Ezetimibe

Ezetimibe is metabolised in the wall of the small intestine to a more potent glucuronide, some of which is further conjugated by the liver. Liver dysfunction increases exposure to the drug [1].

Inhibitors of fasting-induced lipolysis

Acipimox is poorly metabolised. Niacin undergoes saturable first-pass metabolism and is then further extensively metabolised by the liver by a saturable system [19].

Elimination

Statins (HMG-CoA-reductase inhibitors)

The main route of elimination is via the faeces, with small amounts being excreted in the urine, as either metabolites or unchanged drug. Pravastatin is also excreted by the kidneys through tubular secretion [26]. The percentage of pravastatin and simvastatin that is excreted renally is higher than in the other statins: this may be advantageous in obstructive jaundice, where biliary excretion may be impaired. Renal failure has been shown to affect the pharmacokinetics of pravastatin and rosuvastatin [23]. During an episode of HRS, anti-hyperlipidaemic medication should be withheld.

Fibrates

Fenofibrate, ciprofibrate and bezafibrate are excreted primarily in the urine, either as unchanged drug or as metabolites. Gemfibrozil is extensively excreted in bile and its metabolites undergo enterohepatic recycling [19].

Ezetimibe

Ezetimibe undergoes extensive enterohepatic recycling and the amount recycled into the systemic circulation has been estimated at 17–20% [29]. It is excreted primarily in the faeces as unchanged drug.

Inhibitors of fasting-induced lipolysis

Acipimox is excreted primarily in the urine as unchanged drug [19]. Sixty to 76% of a dose of niacin is excreted as unchanged drug and metabolites in the urine [1].

Some relevant adverse effects

Statins (HMG-CoA-reductase inhibitors)

All the statins have been variously implicated in muscle-related adverse drug reactions such as myalgia, myopathy and rhabdomyolysis, which are thought to occur as a direct effect of HMG CoA-reductase inhibition in a dose-dependent manner [30]. There have been fatalities. If patients have increased exposure to a drug due to a reduction in first-pass or subsequent metabolism by hepatocytes, these adverse effects are more likely to occur.

The rate of myopathy with a statin alone in the general population is 0.1–0.5% and 0.2–2.5% with combination therapy. Rhabdomyolysis is very rare at 0.02–0.04%. However, the latter carries a significant morbidity and mortality. In a review of Food and Drug Administration (FDA) reports published in 2002, there were 38 deaths in 631 patients (6.3%) [31]. Pravastatin and fluvastatin have been less frequently implicated in fatal cases of rhabdomyolysis [31]. It is postulated that the more hepatoselective hydrophilic statins, such as pravastatin, are less likely to penetrate muscle cells than are lipophilic statins, and therefore represent a lower risk for myopathy, particularly in the event of an interacting drug increasing their blood levels to within the toxic range [26, 32].

Myopathy and other muscular effects are more common when the statin is co-administered with a second agent likely to be myotoxic or which increases the blood levels of the statin through a drug interaction [33]. One analysis found that in 60% of cases notified to the FDA a second drug was implicated [34]. In August 2001 cerivastatin was withdrawn worldwide following multiple reports of rhabdomyolysis and death, in particular when used with gemfibrozil [35]. The safety of using a statin with other fibrates has been extensively reported on in the medical literature (see Drug Interactions).

Bile acid sequestrants

Colestyramine and colestipol may reduce the absorption of vitamin K and may exacerbate coagulopathy. Monitor INR and PT, especially in active liver disease. They may also cause or worsen constipation, and cause bloating [1].

Fibrates

As fibrates increase the concentration of cholesterol in the bile, there is a theoretical risk of cholelithiasis (gallstones) [1, 19]. All fibrates are reported to cause myopathy and other adverse muscular effects, including rhabdomyolysis [30, 36]. This is more likely to occur in the presence of kidney or liver dysfunction and is more common when the fibrates are used with a statin or other interacting drug. Gemfibrozil, fenofibrate and bezafibrate have been reported to cause a reduction in haemoglobin [1]. Fenofibrate has been reported to reduce fibrinogen levels [19]. This might be significant in patients with thrombocytopenia, coagulopathy, or at risk of a variceal bleed. Pruritus, common in patients with chronic liver disease and often debilitating, has been reported with the fibrates [1].

Ezetimibe

Ezetimibe, either alone or in combination with a statin, rarely causes musculoskeletal effects [1].

Inhibitors of fasting-induced lipolysis

Niacin and acipimox (a niacin analogue) can cause gastric ulceration [1]. They are contraindicated in peptic ulcer disease and should probably be avoided in patients with varices and gastritis. Niacin can reduce the platelet count by 10–15% and should probably be avoided in patients with coagulopathy or thrombocytopenia. Both can cause flushing and pruritus, which is usually transient. That associated with acipimox disappears within the first few days of treatment, and for niacin within the first few weeks. Niacin can cause derangements of blood glucose, necessitating close monitoring of diabetic patients and other patients with potentially erratic blood glucose levels such as those with end-stage liver disease, NASH/metabolic syndrome or acute liver failure. Niacin may augment the effect of vasodilators, increasing the risk of hypotension. This may be problematic in patients using concurrent propranolol, furosemide or spironolactone.

Hepatic adverse effects

Statins (HMG-CoA-reductase inhibitors)

All the statins are reported to cause elevations in transaminases (ALT and AST), either transient or persistent. Rarely, hepatitis may develop. The SPCs of all statins contain a contraindication for their use in the presence of active liver disease or in patients with unexplained, persistent elevations of serum transaminases and any serum transaminase elevation exceeding three times ULN [1]. This may be extremely difficult to interpret in the light of a patient's clinical picture and their need for treatment.

There is controversy about whether or not drugs are more likely to cause hepatotoxicity in patients with liver disease. There is little evidence that statins worsen pre-existing liver disease and hepatocellular damage is very rare, particularly given the high number of prescriptions written worldwide for these drugs [37, 38]. The SPCs note that elevations in liver enzymes occur in between 1/1000 and 1/10 000 patients [1]. Another author notes that the rate of acute hepatic effects for statins is lower than the background rate for the general population [39]. However, this should not be taken to mean that there is no risk. There are many reports of confirmed hepatotoxicity in the literature: hepatitis, jaundice, cholestasis, chronic active hepatitis, fatty liver, cirrhosis and acute liver failure have all been reported. It has also been proposed that statins may 'unmask' latent hepatitis or induce hepatitis [40–42].

The UK Medicines and Healthcare Products Regulatory Agency (MHRA) data show that several deaths have occurred from hepatotoxicity. Most reports of hepatic adverse drug reactions (ADRs) relate to atorvastatin and simvastatin [36]. There are relatively fewer for pravastatin and fluvastatin. However, this may reflect their:

- Relative frequency of use in the UK
- Potential for hepatotoxicity
- Risk of drug interaction-induced toxicity.

There have been very few reports for rosuvastatin, a newer drug to the market.

Russo and Jacobson [38] conclude that there is little evidence to suggest that statins are more hepatotoxic in patients with pre-existing liver disease, and that they may be used for the usual indications with increased monitoring. However, they go on to advise that their use should be avoided in patients with acute liver disease until the acute episode has passed, presumably to avoid the risk of reduced clearance of the drug causing accumulation and an increased risk of toxicity, such as myopathy or rhabdomyolysis.

Several authors agree that, although all lipid-lowering agents can cause transient elevations in transaminases – so-called 'transaminitis' – this may not be true hepatotoxicity, but rather a pharmacodynamic result of the mechanism of action of the drug, to which patients subsequently adapt [14, 43]. One proposed pathway is the leakage of transaminases through the weakened cell membranes of hepatocytes [14]. As AST may be elevated as a result of creatine phosphokinase (CPK) release from muscle injury of any kind, a persistently elevated ALT is a better indicator of a hepatic effect [44]. Measurement of the conjugated and unconjugated fractions of bilirubin may also be useful [2].

The benefit of monitoring LFTs in patients on statins has been questioned by several authors [2, 3, 39, 43]. It is suggested that routine monitoring of LFTs:

- May be meaningless in the absence of a raised bilirubin
- Does not identify those patients at risk of liver damage
- May result in premature cessation of statin therapy, thereby exposing the patient to the risk of a cardiac event
- Is expensive
- May worry the patient unnecessarily [2, 3, 43].

A 2006 review by the National Lipid Association's Statin Safety Assessment Task Force concluded that hepatic function does not appear to be compromised by statin use and that there was no apparent link between elevations in LFTs and the development of liver toxicity. They noted that LFT monitoring may itself be of little value in the absence of other symptoms of liver toxicity, but should be performed for medicolegal reasons, as it is recommended in the product SPCs. The expert group concluded that the use of statins is not contraindicated in chronic and compensated liver disease, but that it is contraindicated in decompensated disease or liver failure [2, 3].

There is disagreement about the wisdom of stopping statins in the event of elevated transaminases, some authors suggesting that the offending statin be switched for another and others advising a 'watch and wait' approach, given the likelihood that the elevated transaminases are transient. A *persistently* elevated ALT (more than three times ULN) should be investigated, as it may indicate an underlying liver pathology [2, 39, 43]. If the elevations are less than three times ULN there is no need to stop the statin [2]. Moreover, statin use may improve elevations in transaminases caused by fatty liver [11, 12]. The National Lipid Association's Statin Safety Assessment Task Force concluded that statins are safe in patients with NASH/NAFLD, provided they are compensated [2, 3].

Despite the controversy about the value of measuring LFTs, it seems prudent to monitor them. LFTs should be checked at baseline, three months, six months and 12 months. Statins may be initiated if the ALT or AST are less than three times ULN. This agrees with the American College of Cardiology/American Heart Association/National Heart, Lung and Blood Institute guidelines [45]. If the patient's transaminases, in particular ALT, rise to three times ULN and remain *persistently* elevated, the dose should be reduced or the drug should be changed for another statin or other class of lipid-lowering agent.

Similarly, the National Lipid Association's Statin Safety Assessment Task Force recommends that LFTs be monitored at baseline, then at 12 weeks or after a dose increase, and periodically thereafter, particularly if the patient has symptoms indicative of liver toxicity. In such patients a full hepatology investigation is warranted (fractionated bilirubin, GGT, ALP, albumin, INR/PT, etc.). Consideration should be given to dose reduction or discontinuation of the statin [2, 3]. In asymptomatic patients, if transaminase levels are more than three times ULN, the test should be repeated. If still more than three times ULN, the patient should have a full liver investigation.

In summary, statins can probably be used safely in liver disease where there is no synthetic dysfunction and even where there is a degree of liver dysfunction provided the appropriate agent is used with a low starting dose (e.g. pravastatin 10 mg or simvastatin 10 mg at night). Patients must be monitored for signs of myopathy. LFTs should be monitored to identify possible hepatotoxicity with persistent elevations in transaminases (more than three times ULN) requiring investigation and discontinuation of the drug.

Bile acid sequestrants

As these drugs are not absorbed, their adverse effects are mainly gastrointestinal in nature and liver adverse effects are not expected.

Fibrates

All lipid-lowering agents, including fibrates, have been reported to cause transient elevations in transaminases, and this may be as a direct result of the mechanism of action of the drug [14]. Brown [46] reports that in a combined study of 20 000 patients the rate of hepatotoxicity was rarely greater than that of placebo. Rarely, bezafibrate causes elevations in ALP, GGT and cholestasis. It can also cause elevations in ALT and AST. Ciprofibrate rarely causes elevations in LFTs and cholestasis. Fenofibrate has been reported to cause elevated transaminases and, rarely, hepatitis. Gemfibrozil rarely causes cholestatic jaundice, raised LFTs and hepatitis [1]. All fibrates increase the cholesterol saturation of bile, leading to an increased risk of cholelithiasis [47]. This characteristic would make fibrates undesirable in obstructive jaundice. The actual occurrence of gallstones appears to be rare, however [1].

Ezetimibe

Ezetimibe rarely causes hepatitis, cholecystitis or cholelithiasis. The rate of elevation of transaminases for ezetimibe is similar to that of placebo, except when it is given with a statin (1.5% vs 1.1% for simvastatin alone, NS) [1, 19].

Inhibitors of fasting-induced lipolysis

Acipimox has not been associated with liver adverse drug reactions [1]. Niacin has been reported to cause transient elevations in transaminases at high doses. This appears to be related to the use of sustained-release (SR) formulations or doses >3 g daily [19, 48, 49]. The SR formulation was designed to reduce the adverse effect of flushing observed with the immediate release (IR) formulation. There are two saturable metabolic pathways, one that produces the metabolite responsible for flushing, and a second whose metabolite is responsible for elevations of transaminases and hepatotoxicity [28]. The IR formulation is metabolised principally via the first route and the rate of flushing can be as high as 100% [50]. The FDA-approved extended-release form (Niaspan® Prolonged Release) is associated with more hepatotoxicity and less flushing, as both routes are used [51]. Hepatitis, focal fatty infiltration of the liver and hepatitis with concurrent haematemesis have all been reported [48]. Acute liver failure has been reported when the SR formulation was substituted for the IR formulation [1]. Patients with Gilbert's syndrome (elevated bilirubin in isolation) may be more prone to the hepatic effects of niacin.

Some relevant drug interactions

Table 11.2 represents only a summary of reported and potential drug interactions. Refer to a comprehensive text on drug interactions or the literature for more information. (Table derived from references 1, 14, 18, 23, 52, 53.)

Those statins more dependent on CYP3A4 metabolism (see Table 11.1) are more likely to exhibit drug interactions. Most clinically impotant drug interactions involving statins result in inhibition of metabolism and an increased risk of toxicity, in particular myotoxicity and rhabdomyolysis. Following the withdrawal of cerivastatin in 2001, it was found that drug interactions were implicated in 60% of reports of rhabdomyolysis to the FDA [34]. The statins have many 'black dot' interactions listed in the BNF, indicating a combination best avoided.

Table 11.2 Summary of major drug interactions

Drug	Mechanism	Potential or reported interacting drugs	Action
Atorvastatin	3A4	Carbamezepine, phenytoin, rifampicin, etc. induce 3A4	
		Imidazoles, grapefruit juice, ciclosporin, macrolides, fluoxetine, etc. inhibit 3A4	
	PGP	Ciclosporin, see above	
	Weak PGP inhibitor	Digoxin, tacrolimus	Monitor tacrolimus levels
Fluvastatin	Unclear ?2D6	Warfarin	Monitor INR
	Unclear	Ciclosporin	
Pravastatin	OATP >> PGP	Ciclosporin	
Rosuvastatin	Unclear	Coumarins	Monitor INR
	Possibly 2C9	Imidazoles, amiodarone (inhibit)	
	OATP	Ciclosporin, itraconazole	
Simvastatin	3A4	As atorvastatin	
	2D6	Coumarins	Monitor INR
	2C9	Imidazoles, amiodarone (inhibit)	
	PGP	See above, ciclosporin	
	PGP inhibitor	Digoxin, tacrolimus	Monitor tacrolimus level
Bezafibrate	Unknown	Ciclosporin, (increased nephrotoxicity)	
	Protein-binding and effects on coagulation	Warfarin, other coumarins	Reduce dose by 50%, monitor INR
	Endocrine effect	Insulin, anti-diabetes drugs	Monitor blood glucose

Table 11.2 Continued

Drug	Mechanism	Potential or reported interacting drugs	Action
Fenofibrate	Unknown Protein-binding and effects on FBC Inhibits 2C9	Ciclosporin (increased nephrotoxicity) Warfarin	Monitor level Reduce dose by 50%, monitor INR
Gemfibrozil	Inhibits OATP, glucuronidation Inhibits 2C8 Weak inhibitor 2C9 (but glucuronide metabolite is strong inhibitor of 2C9) Protein binding and effect on platelets	Fluvastatin Statins Thalindiones (eg. rosiglitazone, repaglinide) Warfarin, other coumarins Potentiate effect of antiplatelet drugs, anticoagulants	Avoid Avoid Reduce dose of anti-coagulant by 50%, monitor INR
Bile acid sequestrants	Inhibits GIT drug absorption	Particularly lipophilic drugs requiring bile salts for absorption	Spaced drug administration
Ezetimibe	Unknown Unknown Additive effect	Warfarin (increased INR) Ciclosporin (raised plasma ezetimibe, ciclosporin) Fibrates, risk of cholelithiasis	Monitor INR Monitor ciclosporin level
Niacin	Use with statins Vasodilation Thrombocytopenia Unknown	Increased risk myopathy, myositis Additive effect with vasodilators Anti-coagulants, anti-platelets Alcohol, high-dose aspirin	Monitor BP Monitor FBC, INR

Other mechanisms for drug interactions are:

- Organic anion transporter protein inhibition (OATP) – transports drugs into hepatocytes
  - Inhibited by ciclosporin, simvastatin
- P-glycoprotein – excretes substrates directly into the gut or renal tubules
  - Inhibition results in increased drug levels (inhibitors include ciclosporin, erythromycin, fenofibrate)
  - Induction results in lower drug levels (inducers include St John's Wort)
- Protein binding
  - Displacement from albumin or other plasma proteins – most statins and fibrates are highly protein bound
- Absorption: usually inhibition of absorption (e.g. bile acid sequestrants)

Many substrates for CYP3A4 are also substrates for P-glycoprotein and OATP.

The *British National Formulary* (BNF) recommends that fibrates or nicotinic acid should not be combined with statins because of the potential for myopathy and rhabdomyolysis with this combination [54]. This is widely discussed in the medical literature. Numerous deaths have been reported and the high mortality associated with concurrent use of cerivastatin and gemfibrozil was partly instrumental in the decision to withdraw cerivastatin from the market in 2001 [34]. It appears that the high mortality in patients using concurrent gemfibrozil and cerivastatin was due to interactions at the level of glucuronidation, CYP2C8 inhibition and OATP inhibition [17, 55].

Fibrates should be used cautiously with warfarin and other coumarins, as the INR may rise significantly. The dose of anticoagulant should be reduced by 50% and then adjusted to INR or PT, using serial measurements [1, 28]. This is in addition to the effect of fibrates on haemoglobin, fibrinogen and antithrombin III, and the interaction may be related to displacement of warfarin from protein-binding site [28]. Fatalities have been reported.

CASE STUDIES

See Appendix 2.1 for details of the following five patient cases.

Patient 1 – Mild hepatitis without cirrhosis

Diagnosis: Non-alcoholic steatohepatitis (NASH)

Patients with NASH frequently have elevated serum cholesterol. In two small studies treatment has been shown to improve serum cholesterol and reduce transaminases, although the value of such treatment needs to be investigated further.

The synthetic and metabolic capacity of this patient's liver is unlikely to be affected by the isolated rise in ALT and AST. Drug handling in this patient is unlikely to be altered, but care must be taken to ensure that they have no signs of cirrhosis, as many patients presenting with this clinical picture can become cirrhotic despite near-normal laboratory tests.

Statins

Although the ALT is slightly higher than three times ULN, a statin could be used with great caution. However, as statins can cause raised ALT and AST, their use may make it difficult to distinguish between iatrogenic elevation of ALT and AST and worsening hepatitis. Monitoring is recommended, as in Hepatic Adverse Effects. The statin should be started at a low dose and increased according to clinical response. There is no specific recommendation in relation to which statin should be used.

Bile acid sequestrants

Colestyramine and colestipol could be used in this patient provided they are not constipated. The INR should be routinely monitored in case vitamin K absorption is inhibited.

Fibrates

Fibrates occasionally cause deranged LFTs: elevated ALT/AST, altered ALP and GGT. Use of a fibrate may make it difficult to distinguish between iatrogenic elevation of ALT and AST and worsening hepatitis.

Ezetimibe

Ezetimibe has caused elevations in transaminases when used with simvastatin, with which it is usually combined.

Inhibitors of fasting-induced lipolysis

Acipimox is not associated with liver adverse drug reactions and should be safe to use. Niacin (nicotinic acid) has been reported to cause transient elevation in transaminases at high doses, as well as more serious hepatic reactions. The SR form could be used with caution. Hepatitis and fibrosis have also been reported.

Summary

A statin could be considered in this patient with appropriate monitoring. Fibrates, niacin or ezetimibe could be used with appropriate monitoring of LFTs. Colestyramine/colestipol and acipimox should be safe to use.

Patient 2 – Cholestasis

Diagnosis: Primary sclerosing cholangitis (PSC)

Secondary hypercholesterolaemia can occur in cholestatic disease. However, medical treatment is usually not indicated.

The synthetic and metabolic capacity of this patient's liver is unlikely to be affected by cholestasis, but consideration needs to be given to:

- Protein-binding (patient has hyperbilirubinaemia)
- Excretion of the drug or metabolites in bile (patient has obstructive jaundice)
- Lipophilicity of the drug (some lipophilic drugs require bile salts for absorption and these would be reduced in cholestasis).

As the patient is taking other medications, potential drug interactions need to be taken into consideration.

Statins

In 2006 the National Lipid Association's Statin Safety Assessment Task Force concluded that chronic liver disease and stable, compensated liver disease are not contraindications to the use of statins [2, 3]. However, statins should be used with caution in this patient for two reasons:

- They are highly excreted in bile and their pharmacodynamic disposition in obstructive cholestasis is unknown.
- They are highly protein bound, and hyperbilirubinaemia may result in increased blood levels of free drug and metabolites through displacement from protein-binding sites.

These effects could result in an increased risk of toxicity.

Statins are also highly lipophilic: if bile salts were required for absorption, this might be reduced.

Pravastatin is less dependent on biliary excretion, a smaller percentage is protein bound, and it is hydrophilic. Therefore, it would be the statin least likely to exhibit altered pharmacodynamics in this patient. However, it has been reported to cause increases in transaminases and should be used with caution and with appropriate monitoring. The drug should be started at a low dose, e.g. 10 mg at night, and then adjusted according to the patient's clinical response.

Bile acid sequestrants

Colestyramine and colestipol could be used in this patient provided there is no constipation. The INR should be routinely monitored in case vitamin K absorption is inhibited. These drugs might have a beneficial effect on the pruritus.

Fibrates

The fibrates are very lipophilic but it is not clear whether they require bile salts for absorption. They are also highly protein bound. Hyperbilirubinaemia may cause displacement from plasma proteins, leading to increased free drug concentrations.

Fenofibrate and bezafibrate are excreted almost entirely in the urine and are more appropriate than gemfibrozil in obstructive jaundice. Gemfibrozil is significantly excreted in bile and undergoes enterohepatic recycling, to which part of its activity is due; this would be reduced by obstructive jaundice. This may lead to a reduction in, or the elimination of, any secondary peaks.

All fibrates can cause an increase in the cholesterol saturation of bile. An increase in gallstone formation has been reported. This is a class effect. The fibrates may cause altered LFTs, including GGT and ALP. Use of a fibrate may make it difficult to distinguish between hepatotoxicity and worsening cholestasis.

Ezetimibe

Ezetimibe is highly lipid soluble but it is not clear whether it requires bile salts for absorption. Part of its activity is due to enterohepatic recycling, which may be reduced by obstructive jaundice. This may lead to a reduction in, or the elimination of, any secondary peaks. It is highly plasma protein bound: hyperbilirubinaemia may cause displacement from plasma proteins, leading to increased free drug concentrations. It has not been reported to cause cholestasis. However, it is generally used with simvastatin, which would not be recommended in this patient (see Statins, above).

Inhibitors of fasting-induced lipolysis

As acipimox and niacin are not highly protein bound and are not lipophilic, cholestasis should not affect their disposition. They are largely excreted in the urine. Neither has been reported to cause cholestasis. Both may cause pruritus, from which this patient suffers.

Drug interactions

Fluvastatin has been reported to interact with rifampicin, causing increased clearance of the statin. Rifampicin is an inducer of the CYP 450 3A4 isoenzyme and may increase the rate of clearance of statins that are substrates for 3A4.

Summary

Pravastatin is the statin of choice in this patient as it is least likely to accumulate, is hydrophilic, and is not highly protein bound. The starting dose should be low and should be increased cautiously. Monitoring of LFTs is required. Colestyramine and colestipol may be considered and may help the patient's pruritus. Niacin and acipimox could be used if the pruritus does not worsen. The fibrates should be avoided because of the risk of gallstone formation. Ezetimibe could be considered alone.

Patient 3 – Compensated cirrhosis

Hyperlipidaemia rarely occurs in cirrhotic patients and cirrhosis may actually protect against atherosclerosis. Despite cirrhosis, this patient is maintaining good hepatocyte function (normal albumin and bilirubin, mildly raised INR) and the metabolic and excretory capacity of the liver should not be significantly reduced. The patient has portal hypertension, so blood flow to the liver will be impaired, which will reduce first-pass metabolism of highly extracted drugs such as statins (extraction ratio >0.7). This will result in greater bioavailability of oral doses of these drugs. It is important to note that the patient could rapidly deteriorate into a state of decompensation where liver function would be markedly affected. Other things to consider are the raised INR and low platelet count (avoid drugs that affect coagulation or cause bleeding); the risk of encephalopathy if liver function decompensates (caution with any drugs causing sedation, constipation, fluid or electrolyte disturbances); and the risk of HRS. During an episode of HRS, anti-hyperlipidaemic medication should be withheld.

Statins

In 2006 the National Lipid Association's Statin Safety Assessment Task Force concluded that chronic liver disease and stable, compensated liver disease are not contraindications to the use of statins, but that they are contraindicated in decompensated disease or liver failure [2, 3]. Although the patient is currently metabolising normally, if decompensation is likely statins are best avoided, as the effects of statin toxicity can be life-threatening.

As the patient has portal hypertension, blood flow through the liver is reduced and the first-pass effect is likely to be lessened, increasing the amount of all statins reaching the systemic circulation. This is not as important for pravastatin, which undergoes less first-pass extraction and is only partly cleared by the liver.

If the patient has stable, compensated disease and a statin is necessary, the drug of choice would be pravastatin. It should be started at a low dose, e.g. 10 mg at night, and increased cautiously. It should be stopped in the event of decompensation.

Bile acid sequestrants

Colestyramine and colestipol could be used provided the patient is not constipated. The INR should be routinely monitored in case vitamin K absorption is inhibited. The patient has thrombocytopenia, which can increase the risk of a bleed. Although the patient has not previously bled, she has one grade 1 varix: a variceal bleed could be serious, particularly in the setting of decompensation.

Fibrates

Fibrates are generally metabolised by the liver and would be expected to be metabolised normally in this patient. However, this might change if the patient's synthetic function deteriorated. Fenofibrate is a prodrug. It is unclear where hydrolysis to the active form takes place. Bezafibrate is only 50% metabolised. Pruritus has been reported with bezafibrate and fenofibrate. Many patients with chronic liver disease have pruritus. Fibrates can cause derangements of LFTs, both cholestatic (GGT and ALP) and hepatitic (AST, ALT). This may be difficult to distinguish from an endogenous change in the patient's liver picture. The fibrates have been reported to cause a reduction in haemoglobin, which might be - significant in this patient, as she has thrombocytopenia and one varix: if decompensation occurred, there would be a risk of a variceal bleed. Fenofibrate can also reduce fibrinogen levels. Fibrates should therefore be avoided in this patient. If a fibrate is absolutely required, bezafibrate could be considered, provided the patient's coagulopathy does not deteriorate.

Ezetimibe

Ezetimibe is only partly metabolised by the liver and should be safe to use alone. However, ezetimibe has caused elevations in transaminases when used with simvastatin, with which it is usually combined. Simvastatin would not be recommended (see Statins, above).

Inhibitors of fasting-induced lipolysis

Acipimox is only partly metabolised and should be safe in this patient. Niacin undergoes extensive first-pass metabolism, which would be reduced due to the decrease in liver blood flow caused by the patient's cirrhosis. Niacin (nicotinic acid) has been reported to cause transient elevations in transaminases at high doses. Hepatitis and fibrosis have also been reported with niacin, usually with the SR once-daily formulation.

Both drugs are gastric irritants and should probably be avoided in patients with varices or a history of variceal bleeding or coagulopathy, or a risk thereof. Niacin can also cause thrombocytopenia. This patient has a varix and would be at risk of a variceal bleed if decompensation occurred. Niacin and acipimox also commonly cause pruritus. They are also vasodilators and may potentiate the effect of drugs that lower blood pressure (spironolactone, propranolol, furosemide), which are used to treat ascites and portal hypertension.

Summary

Statins should be avoided. If absolutely necessary, pravastatin could be used, starting at a low dose and with cautious adjustment according to clinical response. The patient's synthetic liver function should be monitored closely. In the event of the slightest deterioration of function, pravastatin should be stopped immediately. Colestyramine/colestipol should be safe to use but may cause a reduction in vitamin K absorption and increase the risk of a bleed. Constipation might induce encephalopathy. The fibrates should be avoided due to their potential effect on coagulopathy. Ezetimibe should be safe to use alone. Acipimox and niacin are gastric irritants and would be best avoided.

Patient 4 – Decompensated cirrhosis

Hyperlipidaemia rarely occurs in cirrhotic patients. Patients with decompensated disease should not be given medical treatment for hyperlipidaemia: medications should be withheld during the period of decompensation and then reinitiated according to the principles outlined in Case 3 above, when the patient's synthetic function recovers. Note that chronic alcohol use can induce CYP450 enzymes: drugs which are metabolised by this system may be cleared more quickly.

Patient 5 – Acute liver failure

Unnecessary medications should be withheld until the patient's liver function normalises and their pharmaceutical needs are reassessed.

Acknowledgement

My thanks to Professor PA McCormick, Consultant Hepatologist, and Carmel Donnelly, Pharmacist, St.Vincent's University Hospital, Dublin, Ireland.

References

1. www.medicines.org.uk. (2007) Electronic Medicines Compendium.
2. Cohen DE, Anania FA, Chalasani N (2006) An assessment of statin safety by hepatologists. *Am J Cardiol* 97: 77C–81C.

3. McKenney J, Davidson MH, Jacobson TA, Guyton JR (2006) Final conclusions and recommendations of the National Lipid Association Statin Safety Assessment Task Force. *Am J Cardiol* 97: 89C–94C.

4. Jorgensen R, Lindor K, Sartin J, LaRusso N, Wiesner R (1995) Serum lipid and fat-soluble vitamin levels in primary sclerosing cholangitis. *J Clin Gastroenterol* 20: 215–219.

5. Schimming W, Schentke K, Gehrich S, Jaross W, Kobe E (1991) Lipid metabolism disorders in primary biliary cirrhosis (PBC). *Gastroenterol J* 51: 18–21.

6. Chalasani N (2005) Statins and hepatotoxicity: focus on patients with fatty liver. *Hepatology* 41: 690–695.

7. Longo M, Crosignani A, Bettezzati P, *et al.* (2002) Hyperlipidaemic state and cardiovascular risk in primary biliary cirrhosis. *Gut* 51: 265–269.

8. Berzigotti A, Benfiglioli A, Muscari A, *et al.* (2005) Reduced prevalance of ischaemic events and abnormal aupraortic flow patterns in patients with liver cirrhosis. *Liver Int* 25: 331–336.

9. Allocca M, Crosignani A, Gritti A, *et al.* (2006) Hypercholesterolaemia is not associated with early atherosclerotic lesions in primary biliary cirrhosis. *Gut* 55: 1795–1800.

10. Anfossi G, Massucco P, Bonomo K, Trovati M (2004) Prescription of statins to dyslipidemic patients affected by liver diseases: a subtle balance between risks and benefits. *Nutr Metab Cardiovasc Dis* 14: 215–224.

11. Gomez-Dominguez E, Gisbert J, Moreno-Monteagudo J, Garcia-Buey L, Moreno-Otero R (2006) A pilot study of atorvastatin treatment in dyslipemid, non-alcoholic fatty liver patients. *Aliment Pharmacol Ther* 23: 1643–1647.

12. Kiyici M, Gulten M, Gurel S, *et al.* (2003) Ursodeoxycholic acid and atorvastatin in the treatment of nonalcoholic steatohepatitis. *Can J Gastroenterol* 17: 713–718.

13. Fellstrom B (2000) Impact and management of hyperlipidemia posttransplantation. *Transplantation* 70: S51–S58.

14. Corsini A (2003) The safety of HMG-CoA reductase inhibitors in special populations at high cardiovascular risk. *Cardiovasc Drugs Ther* 17: 265–285.

15. Baum C (2001) Weight gain and cardiovascular risk after organ transplantation. *J Parenteral Enteral Nutr* 25: 114–119.

16. Johnston SD, Morrs JK, Cramb R, Gunson BK, Neuberger J (2002) Cardiovascular morbidity and mortality after orthotopic liver transplantation. *Transplantation* 73: 901–906.

17. DeAngelis G (2004) The influence of statin characteristics on their safety and tolerability. *Int J Clin Pract* 58: 945–955.

18. Corsini A, Bellosta S, Davidson MH (2005) Pharmacokinetic interactions between statins and fibrates. *Am J Cardiol* 96: 44K–9K.

19. Dollery C (ed) (1999) *Therapeutic Drugs,* 2nd edn. Edinburgh: Churchill Livingstone.

20. Herman RJ (1999) Drug interactions and the statins. *CMAJ* 161: 1281–1286.

21. Schachter M (2005) Chemical, pharmacokinetic and pharmacodynamic properties of statins: an update. *Fund Clin Pharmacol* 19: 117–125.

22.   Lennernas H (2003) Clinical pharmacokinetics of atorvastatin. *Clin Pharmacokinet* 42: 1141–1160.

23.   Launay-Vacher V, Izzedine H, Deray G (2005) Statins' dosage in patients with renal failure and cyclosporine drug–drug interactions in transplant recipient patients. *Int J Cardiol* 101: 9–17.

24.   Williams D, Feely J (2002) Pharmacokinetic–pharmacodynamic drug interactions with HMG-CoA reductase inhibitors. *Clin Pharmacokinet* 41: 343–370.

25.   Prueksaritanont T, Subramanian R, Fang X, *et al.* (2002) Glucuronidation of statins in animals and humans: a novel mechanism of statin lactonization. *Drug Metab Dispos* 30: 505–512.

26.   Hatanaka T (2000) Clinical pharmacokinetics of pravastatin: mechanisms of pharmacokinetic events. *Clin Pharmacokinet* 39: 397–412.

27.   Garnett WR (1995) Interactions with hydroxymethylglutaryl-coenzyme A reductase inhibitors. *Am J Health Syst Pharm* 52: 1639–1645.

28.   Piepho RW (2000) The pharmacokinetics and pharmacodynamics of agents proven to raise high-density lipoprotein cholesterol. *Am J Cardiol* 86: 35L–40L.

29.   Ezzet F, Krishna G, Wexler DB, Statkevich P, Kosoglou T, Batra VK (2001) A population pharmacokinetic model that describes multiple peaks due to enterohepatic recirculation of ezetimibe. *Clin Ther* 23: 871–885.

30.   Hodel C (2002) Myopathy and rhabdomyolysis with lipid-lowering drugs. *Toxicol Lett* 128: 159–168.

31.   Omar MA, Wilson JP (2002) FDA adverse event reports on statin-associated rhabdomyolysis. *Ann Pharmacother* 36: 288–295.

32.   Vormfelde SV (2001) Safety of statins (hydroxymethyl glutaryl coenzyme a reductase inhibitors): different mechanisms of metabolism and drug transport may have clinical relevance. *Arch Intern Med* 161: 1012–1013.

33.   Ballantyne CM, Corsini A, Davidson MH, *et al.* (2003) Risk for myopathy with statin therapy in high-risk patients. *Arch Intern Med* 163: 553–564.

34.   Bolego C, Baetta R, Bellosta S, Corsini A, Paoletti R (2002) Safety considerations for statins. *Curr Opin Lipidol* 13: 637–644.

35.   Medwatch-Baycol Withdrawal Letter August 2001. Medwatch 2001 Safety Info – Baycol. www.fda.gov/medwatch/safety/2001/Baycol2.htm

36.   Committee for Safety of Medicines (CSM). Adverse Drug Reaction Database. Medicines and Healthcare Regulatory Agency (UK). www.MHRA.gov.uk.

37.   Chalasani N, Aljadhey H, Kesterson J, Murray MD, Hall SD (2004) Patients with elevated liver enzymes are not at higher risk for statin hepatotoxicity. *Gastroenterology* 126: 1287–12.

38.   Russo MW, Jacobson IM (2004) How to use statins in patients with chronic liver disease. *Cleve Clin J Med* 71: 58–62.

39.   Chitturi S, George J (2002) Hepatotoxicity of commonly used drugs: non-steroidal anti-inflammatory drugs, antihypertensives, antidiabetic agents, anticonvulsants, lipid-lowering agents, psychotropic drugs. *Semin Liver Dis* 22: 169–183.

40.   Graziadei IW, Obermoser GE, Sepp NT, Erhart KH, Vogel W (2003) Drug-induced lupus-like syndrome associated with severe autoimmune hepatitis. *Lupus* 12: 409–412.

41. Alla V, Abraham J, Siddiqui J, *et al.* (2006) Auto-immune hepatitis triggered by statins. *J Clin Gastroenterol* 40: 757–761.

42. Pelli N, Setti M, Ceppa P, Toncini C, Indiveri F (2003) Autoimmune hepatitis revealed by atorvastatin. *Eur J Gastroenterol Hepatol* 15: 921–924.

43. Sniderman AD (2004) Is there value in liver function test and creatine phosphokinase monitoring with statin use? *Am J Cardiol* 94: 30F–4F.

44. Dujovne CA (2002) Side effects of statins: hepatitis versus 'ransaminitis'; myositis versus 'CPKitis'. *Am J Cardiol* 89: 1411–1413.

45. Pasternak RC, Smith SC Jr, Bairey-Merz CN, Grundy SM, Cleeman JI, Lenfant C (2002) ACC/AHA/NHLBI Clinical Advisory on the Use and Safety of Statins. *Stroke* 33: 2337–2341.

46. Brown WV (2007) Expert commentary: the safety of fibrates in lipid-lowering therapy. *Am J Cardiol* 99: 19C–21C.

47. Caroli-Bosc FX, Le GP, Pugliese P, *et al.* (2001) Role of fibrates and HMG-CoA reductase inhibitors in gallstone formation: epidemiological study in an unselected population. *Dig Dis Sci* 46: 540–544.

48. Coppola A, Brady PG, Nord HJ (1994) Niacin-induced hepatotoxicity: unusual presentations. *South Med J* 87: 30–32.

49. Pieper JA (2003) Overview of niacin formulations: differences in pharmacokinetics, efficacy, and safety. *Am J Health Syst Pharm* 60(Suppl 2): S9–14.

50. Knodel LC, Talbert RL (1987) Adverse effects of hypolipidaemic drugs. *Med Toxicol* 2: 10–32.

51. McKenney J (2003) Niacin for dyslipidemia: considerations in product selection. *Am J Health Syst Pharm* 60: 995–1005.

52. Stockley I, Baxter K (eds) (2005) *Stockley's Drug Interactions*, 7th edn. London: Pharmaceutical Press.

53. Ogilvie BW, Zhang D, Li W, *et al.* (2006) Glucuronidation converts gemfibrozil to a potent, metabolism-dependent inhibitor of CYP2C8: implications for drug–drug interactions. *Drug Metab Dispos* 34: 191–197.

54. British Medical Association, Royal Pharmaceutical Society of Great Britain (2005) *British National Formulary* No. 50.

55. Shitara Y, Hirano M, Sato H, Sugiyama Y (2004) Gemfibrozil and its glucuronide inhibit the organic anion transporting polypeptide 2 (OATP2/OATP1B1: SLC21A6)-mediated hepatic uptake and CYP2C8-mediated metabolism of cerivastatin: analysis of the mechanism of the clinically relevant drug–drug interaction between cerivastatin and gemfibrozil. *J Pharmacol Exp Ther* 311: 228–236.

12

Scenario 4: Choice of hormone replacement therapy (HRT)

Saw Keng Lee and Sarah Knighton

Introduction

During the menopause a reduction in the levels of oestrogen and proges-terone takes place. This results in women experiencing, among others, vasomotor symptoms (such as hot flushes and night sweats) and vaginal symptoms (dryness, itching and discomfort). In most women, hot flushes are transient and usually resolve within four to five years. However, vaginal symptoms generally persist and can worsen with aging [1]. Hormone replacement therapy (HRT) is therefore used to try to alleviate these symptoms. The benefits of short-term HRT outweigh the risks in the majority of women, especially in those aged under 60 years. Experience in treating women over 65 years with HRT is limited [2].

Owing to the reduction in oestrogen levels during the menopause, an increase in bone loss is seen. However, HRT is generally not recom-mended as first-line therapy for the prophylaxis or treatment of post-menopausal osteoporosis. It should only be used where other therapies are contraindicated, not tolerated, or there is a lack of response. In chronic liver disease HRT may be used first line due to intolerance of other agents, for example bisphosphonates.

HRT is designed to restore the premenopausal physiological state. This is in contrast to oral contraceptive pills, which contain much higher concentrations of oestrogen and progestogen, required to sup-press ovulation. HRT consists of a small dose of oestrogen, given either alone or in combination with a progestogen in women with an intact uterus. The progestogens are given either cyclically or continuously.

Reduction in bone density is an important complication and cause of morbidity in chronic liver disease. This can lead to osteoporosis and osteomalacia with resulting bone fractures, pain, deformity and immo-bility. The problem is greatest in cholestatic liver diseases such as primary biliary cirrhosis (PBC) and primary sclerosing cholangitis (PSC). In postmenopausal women with PBC the rate of bone loss can occur at twice the normal rate (2% vs 1% per year) [3]. Vertebral fracture is the most commonly described fracture in patients with chronic liver disease [4].

Osteoporosis is also common in those on long-term corticosteroid therapy (for example patients with autoimmune hepatitis or coexisting inflammatory bowel disease). Patients with chronic liver disease may also have other risk factors for osteoporosis related to their disease state. These include vitamin D deficiency, excessive alcohol consumption, poor diet, physical inactivity and low body mass index. Oestrogen deficiency in the postmenopausal stage further increases the risk.

HRT has been shown to be effective in reducing bone loss and fractures in postmenopausal women. It inhibits bone resorption and stimulates new bone formation [5]. When HRT is given in the first five to ten years of menopause the long-term risk of osteoporotic fractures is halved [5].

The risks and benefits of HRT should be carefully assessed on an individual basis. This is particularly important in women with predisposing risk factors, such as a personal or family history of deep vein thrombosis or pulmonary embolism, severe varicose veins, obesity or prolonged bed-rest [2], because HRT increases the risk of venous thromboembolism and stroke. HRT has also been observed to increase the risk of gallbladder disease, breast cancer and endometrial cancer. It is recommended that the minimum effective dose should be used for the shortest period of time, with treatment being reviewed at least once a year [2].

In women with an intact uterus a progestogen should be added to reduce the risk of endometrial hyperplasia and possible transformation to cancer. However, the addition of a progestogen should be weighed against the increased risk of breast cancer associated with its use.

Summary

The use of HRT is generally cautioned in liver disease because of concern over its potential to provoke or worsen cholestasis. This is based on early experience with oral contraceptive pills that contained higher doses of the less degradable synthetic oestrogen ethinylestradiol. However, several studies have demonstrated the safety and efficacy of HRT in patients with chronic liver disease, in particular those with PBC and viral hepatitis. HRT may be particularly beneficial in patients with PBC owing to the high prevalence of osteoporosis in this population.

Consensus guidelines for the management of osteoporosis in patients with chronic liver disease recommend transdermal HRT (containing oestradiol 50 µg/day plus progestogen in women with an intact uterus) in combination with oral calcium and vitamin D supplementation, as first-line therapy.

The pharmacokinetics of oestrogen and progestogen can be significantly altered in patients with liver disease. Oestrogens and progestogens are highly lipophilic, therefore oral absorption may be reduced in patients with cholestasis. Both oestrogen and progestogen undergo extensive first-pass metabolism in the liver. However, newer HRT preparations usually contain either a readily degradable oestradiol or conjugated equine oestrogens. Amongst the progestogens, norethisterone derivatives have more of an effect on liver metabolism than do the progesterone derivatives [6].

In patients with portal hypertension impaired blood flow to the liver may decrease the first-pass metabolism of oral oestrogen and progestogen, with a resulting increase in bioavailability. In addition, their binding and distribution may be affected in patients with low albumin, as they are highly protein bound. However, the clinical significance of these changes is unknown. It would therefore be prudent to monitor the patient closely for efficacy and safety during treatment.

The metabolites of both oestrogen and progestogen are excreted into the bile. Oestrogen metabolites undergo extensive enterohepatic circulation before being eliminated in the urine. Progestogens do not undergo enterohepatic circulation and their metabolites are excreted mainly in faeces and urine.

In patients with cholestasis, biliary excretion may be impaired, reducing the overall drug exposure, which could lead to decreased efficacy. However, such effect has not been reported in the clinical studies involving oral HRT. Studies have also suggested that women who are already jaundiced are most at risk of increased cholestasis with HRT.

The transdermal or subcutaneous routes are more favourable as they avoid first-pass metabolism. However, subcutaneous implants may result in prolonged endometrial stimulation, even after discontinuation. Topical therapy may be used to provide symptomatic relief of vaginal symptoms.

A small increase in the risk of gallbladder disease has been associated with the use of HRT. Studies have shown that preparations containing oestrogen alone are associated with a greater risk than combination oestrogen/progestogen therapy. The formulation used is important, with transdermal preparations considered safer.

Before starting HRT patients should be assessed individually considering their risk of osteoporosis, the current status of their liver disease, and any other coexisting medical risks. They should also be assessed for any history, including family history, of jaundice. The risks and potential benefits of treatment should be carefully explained.

Liver enzymes and serum bilirubin should be measured before treatment is commenced to indicate the degree of cholestasis. These parameters should then be closely monitored, with treatment being stopped if a significant increase is seen. The optimum duration of treatment has yet to be defined, but it is recommended that the minimum effective dose should be used for the shortest period.

Unless otherwise stated, all pharmacokinetic data originate from standard reference sources [28–32] and apply to adults only.

Pharmacokinetics

See Table 12.1 for a summary of the pharmacokinetics of HRT in adults.

Absorption

Orally administered oestrogens are completely absorbed from the gastrointestinal tract, with peak plasma concentrations occurring within one-half to five hours. Bioavailability is low due to extensive first-pass metabolism in the small intestinal mucosa and liver. Many of the commercially available oral preparations of HRT contain formulations of oestrogens that release slowly over several hours.

Orally administered progestogens are also completely absorbed from the gastrointestinal tract, with peak serum levels occurring within one to five hours. The bioavailability of progestogens varies greatly.

Oestrogens and progestogens can also be administered by subcutaneous implants or transdermally, thereby avoiding first-pass metabolism. These routes cause a slower and more prolonged increase in plasma concentrations of hormones compared to oral administration. HRT is usually given transdermally or orally, although topical gels for vaginal use are also available.

Tibolone is rapidly and extensively absorbed. The extent of presystemic metabolism, and hence bioavailability, is not known.

Raloxifene is rapidly absorbed following oral administration. It then undergoes extensive first-pass metabolism (presystemic glucuronidation).

Distribution

Oestrogens and progestogens are widely distributed in the body and are found in higher concentrations in the sex hormone target organs. Once absorbed, oestrogens and progestogens are transported in the blood to the liver, mainly bound to plasma proteins or sex hormone-binding globulin (oestrogens only). A small proportion (1–5%) is transported as free steroid (unbound).

Data on the distribution of tibolone are limited. It is transported in the blood to the liver bound to plasma proteins (96%), most likely albumin.

Raloxifene is distributed extensively throughout the body, with the volume of distribution being dose dependent. It is highly protein bound (98–99%) to plasma proteins, including albumin.

Metabolism

Orally administered oestrogens undergo extensive first-pass metabolism in the small intestinal mucosa and liver by a hydroxysteroid dehydrogenase. These metabolites are converted to glucuronide and sulphate conjugates. Unlike ethinylestradiol, oestradiol is readily oxidised to oestrone and oestriol.

Progestogen metabolism is not as widely documented, but it also undergoes first-pass metabolism. The major route of liver metabolism is via hydroxylation, with subsequent conjugation and elimination. The clinical significance of many progestogen metabolites is unknown.

Tibolone is rapidly broken down into three active metabolites, two having oestrogen-like activity, the third having progestagenic and androgen-like activity. *In-vitro* studies have suggested that tibolone may undergo tissue-selective local metabolism. The relevance of this is, however, unknown [7].

Elimination

After metabolism, conjugates of oestrogens and progestogens are excreted into the bile. Following subsequent biliary secretion into the intestine, the oestrogen metabolites undergo hydrolysis, followed by reabsorption. This is known as enterohepatic circulation. This means that there is a constant circulating reservoir for the formation of the active oestrogen metabolites. Oestrogen metabolites and conjugates are eliminated in the urine.

Table 12.1 Pharmacokinetics of HRT in adults

Drug	Bio-availability	T_{max} (hrs)	Lipophilicity	Protein binding %	Half-life (hrs)
Drospirenone (oral)	76–85%	1	–	97	36–42
Estradiol (oral)	Low	0.5–5	High	97–99	2–16
Estradiol (transdermal)	–	36–42	–	97–99	2–16
Medroxyprogesterone acetate (oral)	Low	2–6	High	94	30
Norethisterone acetate (oral)	64%	0.5–2	High	90–95	6–11
Norethisterone acetate (transdermal)	–	37–48	–	90–95	6–15
Raloxifene	2%	28	–	>95	28
Tibolone	Unknown	1.5–4	High	96	–

% excreted unchanged in urine	% Biliary excreted	Metabolism	Active metabolites
Mainly excreted as metabolites	Excreted as metabolites in faeces	Extensive metabolism	The two major metabolites are pharmacologically inactive
Mainly excreted as metabolites	40% Undergoes enterohepatic circulation	Extensive first-pass metabolism in gut and liver Reduction, hydroxylation and conjugation to form both glucuronide and sulfate conjugates	Oesterone Oestriol
Mainly excreted as metabolites	40% Undergoes enterohepatic circulation	No first-pass effect Reduction, hydroxylation and conjugation to form both glucuronide and sulfate conjugates	Oesterone Oestriol
<5%	–	Extensively metabolized Undergoes hydroxylation, de-esterification, transesterification, demethylation, conjugation, reduction	Unknown
Low Excreted mainly as metabolites	Excreted as metabolites in faeces	First-pass metabolism Reduction then conjugated with glucuronide or sulfate	Norethisterone 5α-dihydronorethisterone Tetrahydronorethisterone
Low Mainly excreted as metabolites in urine	Excreted as metabolites in faeces	Reduction then conjugated with glucuronide or sulfate	Norethisterone 5α-dihydronorethisterone Tetrahydronorethisterone
< 0.2% Less than 6% excreted as conjugates	>90% Undergoes enterohepatic circulation Excreted as metabolites in faeces	Extensive first-pass metabolism Glucuronide conjugates formed	Unknown
Excreted as metabolites (40%)	Excreted as metabolites in faeces (60%)	Extensive metabolism in liver and intestine	3β-hydroxytibolone 3α-hydroxytibolone Tibolone-4-ene

Progestogens do not undergo enterohepatic circulation. Metabolites are excreted in the faeces and urine. Only a small proportion of a dose of progestogen is excreted unchanged in the urine.

Tibolone does not undergo enterohepatic circulation. Excretion occurs mainly via the faecal route, with urinary excretion accounting for the remainder.

Raloxifene undergoes enterohepatic circulation, allowing the maintenance of plasma levels and giving it a longer half-life. The majority of a dose of raloxifene and its metabolites are excreted via biliary excretion, with elimination in the faeces. Only a small proportion is excreted via the urine [8].

Some relevant adverse effects

Hepatotoxicity

Because the dose of oestrogens and progestogens used in HRT products is low, the majority of women experience no adverse effects on liver function. Occasionally hepatic changes such as cholestatic jaundice, vascular complications and enlargement of haemangiomas have occurred. See the Clinical studies and Case reports sections below for further details.

Biliary effects

An increased risk of gallbladder disease has been associated with the use of HRT [9].

Gastrointestinal effects

Abdominal pain and bloating have been associated with the use of HRT.

Some relevant drug interactions

Concomitant use of substances known to induce cytochrome P450 enzymes, in particular CYP3A4, may increase the metabolism of oestrogens and progestogens, leading to reduced effect and changes in the uterine bleeding profile. Conversely, drugs that inhibit these enzymes may reduce metabolism, leading to a higher exposure. The clinical significance of this is, however, unknown.

In clinical practice drug interactions are relatively uncommon in women using HRT, owing to the low doses of oestrogen and progestogen used.

There is no evidence that tibolone causes enzyme induction. In theory, substances that induce cytochrome P450 may affect the metabolism of tibolone and lead to reduced activity. However, no interactions between tibolone and other medicines have been reported in clinical practice [7].

No clinically important interactions have been reported when raloxifene is co-administered with several groups of drugs, including analgesics [8].

Clinical studies and case reports

Women without liver disease

Two small studies have examined the effect of HRT on liver function tests in healthy women. The women had regular assessment of their liver function tests during therapy. Hepatotoxicity and cholestasis were not observed [10, 11].

Observational data have suggested that HRT users may have a better profile of liver function tests. One randomised placebo-controlled study involving 50 women with type 2 diabetes demonstrated that HRT containing oestradiol 1 mg and norethisterone 0.5 mg significantly improved serum concentrations of liver enzymes. The authors hypothesised that this might be due to HRT causing a reduction in liver fat content. However, further work in this area to understand the significance and mechanisms by which this occurs was recommended [12].

HRT has also been shown to cause favourable changes in serum lipid levels in normal postmenopausal women [13]. This effect could be particularly beneficial in women with cholestatic liver disease who may have elevated serum cholesterol.

Women with cholestatic liver disease

Many of the studies looking at the use of HRT in liver disease involve women with PBC, owing to the high prevalence of osteoporosis in this population (approximately 30%) [14]. In a small retrospective study of postmenopausal women with PBC, 16 received HRT. This was shown to cause a significant increase in bone mineral density in the lumbar spine compared to the untreated group at one-year follow-up. No worsening of cholestasis was observed in the HRT group [15]. However, the dose, form and duration of HRT therapy used in this study were not consistent. Another similar study involving ten women with PBC (nine with osteoporosis and one with osteopenia) who received HRT for two years also found that HRT was safe and effective [16].

The findings of these studies were confirmed by a longer retrospective study involving 46 women with PBC. HRT significantly lowered the rate of bone loss compared to age-matched untreated women. This study had a much longer follow-up period (4.8 ± 0.4 years), but also demonstrated that HRT is safe and effective in PBC [17]. However, as with the previous studies, the HRT preparations used were not standardised.

The effect of ethinylestradiol 50 µg daily on liver function tests was examined in five women with PBC. These patients had been previously exposed to various HRT preparations (oestrogen or an oestrogen–progestogen combination). Three of the women, who had normal or near-normal serum bilirubin before treatment, tolerated HRT well. However, the remaining two, who were profoundly jaundiced (with serum bilirubins of 193 µmol/L and 365 µmol/L, respectively) before treatment, experienced a further increase in serum bilirubin levels two to three months after starting treatment. A decrease in bilirubin levels occurred in both patients upon withdrawal of ethinylestradiol [18].

The findings of this study suggest that women who are already jaundiced at the initiation of HRT are most at risk of increased bilirubin levels and cholestasis. In view of this it would seem sensible that, as well as assessing bilirubin levels prior to treatment, women who want to take HRT should also be assessed for any history (including family history) of jaundice. This will include specific defects in bilirubin excretion, such as intrahepatic cholestasis of pregnancy or familial conjugated hyperbilirubinaemia, which may worsen cholestasis.

The safety and efficacy of transdermal HRT was examined in a one-year controlled trial involving 42 postmenopausal women with PBC [19]. They were treated with calcium and vitamin D either alone or combined with HRT. A total of 21 women received HRT (13 received combination oestradiol and norethisterone, with the remaining eight receiving oestradiol alone). The follow-up period was one year. Those receiving HRT plus calcium and vitamin D showed improved lumbar spine bone mineral density compared to the group receiving calcium and vitamin D alone. No significant change in liver function tests was observed. In particular, worsening of cholestasis was not seen despite nine of the 21 patients receiving HRT having raised serum bilirubin levels (mean bilirubin 29.6 ± 4.9 µmol/L) prior to the start of treatment and one being clinically jaundiced (65 µmol/L). The effect of HRT on this particular patient's bilirubin level was unfortunately not discussed further in this study [19].

A similar study involving 18 postmenopausal women with PBC looked at the safety and efficacy of transdermal HRT over a two-year period. The women were randomised to receive calcium and alfacalcidol either alone or in combination with HRT (oestradiol and medroxyprogesterone). A significant increase in bone mineral density in the lumbar spine and femoral neck was seen in the group receiving HRT [14]. One patient was withdrawn from the study because of a significant rise in AST (three times above baseline) and ALT (five times above baseline) levels. No change in ALP or bilirubin was observed. Upon withdrawal of treatment AST and ALT returned to baseline levels within three months. The authors concluded that, in the absence of other factors, oestrogen therapy was the likely cause of this [14].

Women with viral hepatitis

The safety of transdermal HRT (oestradiol 50 µg/day, norethisterone 250 µg/day for 14 days per 28-day cycle) was investigated in 81 postmenopausal women with chronic hepatitis B and/or C. The liver enzymes of these women remained unaffected after five years of treatment. In those with signs of hepatomegaly or steatosis of the liver, HRT actually seemed to slow the progression toward liver fibrosis [20]. A similar result was also seen in a retrospective study of women with hepatitis C receiving HRT. This study suggested that HRT appeared to be associated with a protective effect against the progression of fibrosis [21]. This has also been demonstrated in an animal study which showed that endogenous and exogenous oestrogens have a protective effect on liver fibrosis [22]. A positive effect of oestrogens on liver cirrhosis, potentially linked to the antioxidant properties of oestradiol, has also been suggested [23].

Risk of gallbladder disease

An increased risk of gallbladder disease has been associated with the use of HRT. This is believed to be due to oestrogens and progestogens causing an increase in levels of biliary cholesterol while reducing the relative level of bile acids. This leads to an increase of cholesterol saturation in bile, predisposing to gallstone formation. Gallbladder contractility may also be affected [9].

Several studies have tried to quantify the risk of gallbladder disease in women receiving HRT. The Heart and Oestrogen/Progestin Replacement Study found that gallbladder disease occurred in 3% of patients who received HRT, compared to 2.2% of those who received placebo [9]. Two Women's Health Initiative trials showed a greater risk of gallbladder disease or surgery with oestrogen alone than with oestrogen and progestogen preparations. In women who were receiving oestrogen alone, there were 78 events per 10 000 person-years, compared to 55 events per 10 000 person-years in women receiving combined preparations [9].

The formulation of HRT used may also affect the risk of gallbladder disease. One small study involving 17 patients compared transdermal oestradiol (100 µg daily) to oral oestradiol (2 mg daily). It found that, unlike oral therapy, transdermal oestradiol did not induce lithogenic bile or increase the risk of gallstone formation [24]. Oral oestrogen therapy causes a more pronounced increase in oesterone levels than does transdermal administration. This increase correlates with an increase in the cholesterol saturation index, which can lead to gallstone formation [9, 24, 25]. This finding is supported by other studies showing that transdermal oestrogen appears to have less of an effect on liver function than oral administration [24, 25]. This is thought to be because transdermal oestrogens more closely mimic physiological oestrogen/oestradiol ratios. Therefore, transdermal therapy may be advantageous in patients with cholestatic liver disease, particularly PBC, in which gallstones are common.

Raloxifene

Raloxifene undergoes extensive first-pass metabolism to glucuronide conjugates. It is then eliminated by biliary excretion. The pharmacokinetics of raloxifene have been studied in patients with mild hepatic impairment (Child–Pugh class A) and concentrations were found to be approximately 2.5 times higher than in controls, correlating with the patient's bilirubin concentration [8].

Recommendations on the use of HRT in liver disease

Williams *et al.* [26] have recommended that HRT should be considered '…in all women with chronic liver disease who are postmenopausal, have primary or secondary amenorrhoea, or have had oophorectomy'. Transdermal therapy is preferred. Serum bilirubin and liver enzymes should be measured before treatment is initiated to indicate the degree of cholestasis. These tests should then be repeated one month after treatment is started. If the serum GGT and ALP have not increased by more than 100%, and the serum bilirubin has remained normal, then treatment can be continued. Liver function tests should then be monitored every six months. On the other hand, if the serum GGT and ALP have increased by more than 100%, or if serum bilirubin has risen, liver function tests should be checked every month for at least three months. Treatment should be stopped if a significant increase is seen [26].

Consensus guidelines on the management of osteoporosis associated with chronic liver disease recommend oral calcium and vitamin D supplementation plus transdermal HRT as first-line therapy for women with established osteoporosis. Transdermal oestradiol should be used at a dose of 50 µg/day (equivalent to 2 mg daily of oral oestradiol). This should be given in combination with a progestogen in women with an intact uterus [4]. Oral bisphosphonates should be avoided in cirrhotic patients who may have portal hypertension and oesophageal varices because of their potential to precipitate a variceal bleed [4, 27].

The risks and benefits of HRT should be assessed for each patient by taking into consideration individual risk factors and the severity of their liver disease. These should be discussed with the patient before the initiation of therapy. Liver function tests should be monitored before treatment is begun, and then during treatment as appropriate. The optimum duration of therapy has yet to be defined in liver patients. The minimum effective dose should be used for the shortest period. The decision to continue treatment must be made on an individual basis, in view of the risks associated with use of HRT.

CASE STUDIES

See Appendix 1 for full details of the following patient cases.

Patient 1 – Mild hepatitis without cirrhosis

The synthetic and metabolic capacity of this patient's liver is unlikely to be affected by the isolated rise in ALT, and drug handling is unlikely to be altered. It is important to ensure that the patient has no signs of cirrhosis, as many diseases that present with this clinical picture can be cirrhotic despite near-normal laboratory tests.

- In the treatment of menopausal symptoms the benefits of short-term HRT may outweigh the risks, especially in this patient, who is under 60 years of age.
- Apart from protection against osteoporosis, HRT is also associated with favourable changes in serum lipid levels in postmenopausal women. This may be helpful in this patient, who has fatty liver disease.
- HRT has also been associated with a protective effect against the progression of fibrosis. However, this has yet to be confirmed in a large randomised controlled trial.
- The best choice for this patient would be HRT via the transdermal route, as this avoids first-pass metabolism. Although the synthetic and metabolic capacity of the liver is unlikely to be affected, oral therapy should be avoided.
- Ethinylestradiol is not recommended as it is less degradable. Therefore, an oestradiol-containing preparation should be used.
- A combination product containing oestrogen and progestogen should be used if the patient has an intact uterus.
- The lowest effective dose for the shortest period of time should be used.
- Liver function tests should be measured before treatment is started. These should then be monitored closely during treatment. Treatment should be stopped if a significant change occurs.

Patient 2 – Cholestasis

The synthetic and metabolic capacity of this patient's liver is unlikely to be affected by cholestasis. However, consideration needs to be given to protein binding (patient has hyperbilirubinaemia); excretion of the drug or metabolites in bile (patient has cholestasis); and the lipophilicity of the drug (some lipophilic drugs require bile salts for absorption, and these would be reduced in cholestasis).

- Loss of bone density is an important complication and particularly common in cholestatic liver diseases such as PSC. Therefore, HRT would be beneficial in this patient.
- Although the synthetic and metabolic capacity of the liver is unlikely to be affected, oral therapy should be avoided. Oestrogens and progestogens are highly lipophilic, therefore absorption may be reduced.
- Oestrogens undergo enterohepatic circulation. As this patient is cholestatic, biliary excretion may be impaired. This may reduce the overall exposure to the drug, which could lead to decreased efficacy. However, this was not reported as a problem in the clinical studies involving oral HRT that have been carried out in similar patient populations.

- Ethinylestradiol is not recommended as it is less degradable. Therefore, an oestradiol-containing preparation should be used.
- A combination product containing oestrogen and progestogen should be used if the patient has an intact uterus.
- As this patient has cholestasis they may be at a higher risk of HRT causing a further increase in bilirubin levels and worsening cholestasis. Liver function tests should be measured before treatment is started, and be monitored closely during treatment. Treatment should be stopped if a significant change occurs.
- The patient should be checked for any skin sensitivity before using the transdermal patch. Any skin reaction may worsen pruritus already suffered by the patient.
- The lowest effective dose for the shortest period of time should be used.

Patient 3 – Compensated cirrhosis

Despite cirrhosis, this patient is maintaining good hepatocyte function (normal albumin and bilirubin, mildly raised INR) and the metabolic and excretory capacity of the liver should not be significantly reduced. The patient has portal hypertension, so blood flow to the liver will be impaired, which will reduce the first-pass metabolism of highly extracted drugs (extraction ratio >0.7). This will result in greater bioavailability of oral doses of these drugs. It is important to note that the patient could rapidly deteriorate into a state of decompensation where liver function would be markedly affected.

Other things to consider are the raised INR and low platelet count, the risk of encephalopathy if the liver function decompensates, and the risk of hepatorenal syndrome.

- Oral therapy should be avoided as oestrogens and progestogens undergo extensive first-pass metabolism. Therefore, exposure to the drug would be increased, with a resulting increased risk of hepatotoxicity.
- The best choice for this patient would be HRT via the transdermal route, as this avoids first-pass metabolism.
- Ethinylestradiol is not recommended as it is less degradable. Therefore, an oestradiol-containing preparation should be used.
- A combination product containing oestrogen and progestogen should be used if the patient has an intact uterus.
- The lowest effective dose for the shortest period of time should be used.
- Liver function tests should be measured before treatment is started. These should then be monitored closely during treatment. Treatment should be stopped if a significant change occurs.

- The patient should be checked for skin sensitivity before using the transdermal patch. Any skin reaction may worsen pruritus already suffered by the patient.

Patient 4 – Decompensated cirrhosis

HRT (oral and transdermal) should not be initiated or continued in patients with decompensated cirrhosis. The hepatocyte damage is irreversible and can only worsen over time. The significant reduction in metabolic capacity and reduction in hepatic blood flow will lead to drug accumulation, with consequent increased risk of hepatotoxicity. There is also the potential to worsen the cholestatic picture in this patient, who is already profoundly jaundiced.

Patient 5 – Acute liver failure

There is no place for HRT in a 16-year-old girl. HRT is also otherwise contraindicated in acute liver failure. The rapid hepatocyte damage has led to poor synthetic function and a significant reduction in the ability of the liver to metabolise the drug. This will only result in drug accumulation and hence added hepatotoxicity in acute liver failure.

Acknowledgements

We are grateful to Caroline Burgess, Medicines Information at King's College Hospital for her contribution to the literature search and her determination in gathering articles that have proved challenging to obtain. We would also like to thank Dr Astrid Scalori, Specialist Hepatology Registrar, who kindly read the chapter with interest and offered valuable advice.

References

1. Grady D (2006) Management of menopausal symptoms. *N Engl J Med* 355: 2338–2347.
2. Hormone Replacement Therapy. *British National Formulary*, September 2006.
3. Eastell R, Dickson ER, Hodgson SF, *et al.* (1991) Rates of vertebral bone loss before and after liver transplantation in women with primary biliary cirrhosis. *Hepatology* 14: 296–300.
4. Collier JD, Ninkovic M, Compston JE (2002) Guidelines on the management of osteoporosis associated with chronic liver disease. *Gut* 50 (Suppl I): S1–9.

5. Riggs BL, Melton LJ (1993) The prevention and treatment of osteoporosis. *N Engl J Med* 327: 620–627.
6. Kuhl H (1990) Pharmacokinetics of oestrogens and progestogens. *Maturitas* 12(3): 171–197.
7. Livial. Summary of Product Characteristics. Organon Lab Ltd. Available at http: medicines.org.uk. Updated 19 June 2006.
8. Evista. Summary of Product Characteristics. Eli Lilly and Company Ltd. Available at http://medicines.org.uk. Updated 19 January 2007.
9. Kalala S, Krishna M, Shah R, *et al.* (2006) Postmenopausal hormone replacement therapy and the risks of calculous gallbladder disease. *Clin Geriatr* 14: 25–29.
10. Moore B, Paterson M, Sturdee D (1987) Effect of oral hormone replacement therapy on liver function tests. *Maturitas* 9: 7–15.
11. Darj E, Axelsson O, Carlstrom K, *et al.* (1993) Liver metabolism during treatment with oestradiol and natural progesterone. *Gynecol Endocrinol* 7: 111–114.
12. McKenzie J, Fisher BM, Jaap AJ, *et al.* (2006) Effects of HRT on liver enzyme levels in women with type 2 diabetes: a randomised placebo-controlled trial. *Clin Endocrinol* 65: 40–44.
13. Kable WT, Gallagher JC, Nachtigall L, *et al.* (1990) Lipid changes after hormone replacement therapy for menopause. *J Reprod Med* 35: 512–518.
14. Ormarsdóttir S, Mallmin H, Naessén T, *et al.* (2004) An open, randomised, controlled study of transdermal hormone replacement therapy on the rate of bone loss in primary biliary cirrhosis. *J Intern Med* 256: 63–69.
15. Crippin JS, Jorgensen RA, Dickson ER, *et al.* (1994) Hepatic osteodystrophy in primary biliary cirrhosis: Effects of medical treatment. *Am J Gastroenterol* 89: 47–50.
16. Olsson R, Mattsson LA, Obrant K, *et al.* (1999) Oestrogen–progestogen therapy for low bone mineral density in primary biliary cirrhosis. *Liver* 19: 188–192.
17. Narayanan Menon KV, Angulo P, Boe GM, *et al.* (2003) Safety and efficacy of oestrogen therapy in preventing bone loss in primary biliary cirrhosis. *Am J Gastroenterol* 98: 889–892.
18. Guattery JM, Faloon WW (1987) Effect of oestradiol upon serum enzymes in primary biliary cirrhosis. *Hepatology* 7: 737–742.
19. Pereira SP, O'Donohue J, Moniz C, *et al.* (2004) Transdermal hormone replacement therapy improves vertebral bone density in primary biliary cirrhosis: results of a 1-year controlled trial. *Aliment Pharmacol Ther* 19: 563–570.
20. Rinaldi M, Cagancci A, Pansini FE, *et al.* (2005) Neutral effect of prolonged transdermal hormone therapy on liver function of postmenopausal women with chronic active hepatitis. *Menopause* 12: 619–622.
21. Di Martino V, Lebray P, Myers RP, *et al.* (2004) Progression of liver fibrosis in women infected with hepatitis C: Long-term benefit of oestrogen exposure. *Hepatology* 40: 1426–1433.
22. Yasuda M, Shimizu I, Shiba M, *et al.* (1999) Suppressive effects of oestradiol on dimethylnitrosamine-induced fibrosis of the liver in rats. *Hepatology* 29: 719–727.

23. Shimizu I (2003) Impact of oestrogens on the progression of liver disease. *Liver Intern* 23: 63–69.

24. Van Erpecum KJ, Van Berge Henegouwen GP, Verschoor L, *et al.* (1991) Different hepatobiliary effects of oral and transdermal oestradiol in post-menopausal women. *Gastroenterology* 100: 482–488.

25. Uhler ML, Marks JW, Voigt BJ, *et al.* (1998) Comparison of the impact of transdermal versus oral oestrogens on biliary markers of gallstone formation in postmenopausal women. *J Clin Endocrinol Metab* 83: 410–414.

26. Williams R, O'Donohue J (1997) Hormone replacement therapy in women with liver disease. *Br J Obstet Gynaecol* 104: 1–3.

27. Hay JE, Guichelaar MMJ (2005) Evaluation and management of osteoporosis in liver disease. *Clin Liver Dis* 9: 747–766.

28. Dollery C (ed) (1999) *Therapeutic Drugs*, 2nd edn. Edinburgh: Churchill Livingstone.

29. Sweetman S (ed) (2005) *Martindale: The Complete Drug Reference*, 34th edn. London: Pharmaceutical Press.

30. McEvoy GK (ed) (2006) *AHFS Drug Information*. Bethesda, MA: American Society of Health-System Pharmacists.

31. Hutchison TA, Shahan DR, Anderson ML (eds) (2007) Drugdex System Internet version Micromedex Inc. Greenwood Village, Colorado (accessed 8 March 2007).

32. Baxter I (ed) (2005) *Stockley's Drug Interactions*, 7th edn. London: Pharmaceutical Press.

13

Scenario 5: Choice of contraceptive

Aileen Parke

Introduction

Women with severe liver disease are considered unlikely to conceive or become pregnant, as up to 50% suffer from amenorrhea due to advanced reproductive age, metabolic abnormalities or hormonal disturbances. Menstrual abnormalities, such as oligomenorrhoea and metrorrhagia, are also often associated with infertility in women with chronic liver disease (CLD) [1]. The interaction between the liver and contraceptives has implications for women with liver disease, and the methods available should be carefully considered [2].

Various methods of contraception are available and may be considered in women with liver disease. Permanent methods, e.g. tubal ligation, may be suitable for some patients, but reversible contraceptive methods are usually preferred. Hormone methods are based on progestogens alone (POC) or in combination with ethinylestradiol (EE), as an oral preparation (COC) or a patch, and provide 99% efficacy in compliant women. POCs are available as an oral preparation (POP) or as long-acting systems, such as intramuscular depot medroxyprogesterone (DMPA), progestogen-only implants (IMP) and levonorgestrel-releasing intrauterine devices (LNG-IUD). Non-hormonal methods include the copper intrauterine device (Cu-IUD) and barrier methods such as condoms or a diaphragm. The barrier methods have lower efficacy rates, ranging between 80% and 95% compared to 98–99% for the other methods [2,3].

Summary

The preferred choice of contraception for any woman with liver disease would be a barrier method, thereby avoiding any interaction with the liver and preventing side effects. This method is especially useful in viral hepatitis to reduce the risk of transmission. IUDs may be used in women with cholestatic or mild hepatitic liver disease, but should be used with caution in women with cirrhosis and avoided in those with ascites or coagulopathy because of the risks of infection and bleeding. Oestrogen-containing contraceptives should be avoided in all hepatitic liver disease, as they may worsen the condition and are associated with a higher level of side effects in women with certain types of pre-existing liver disease. Oestrogens can be used in most cholestatic conditions but should be reviewed if the condition changes or progresses. Progestogen-only preparations are generally safe in women with liver disease but should be avoided in patients with decompensated cirrhosis, as their metabolism may be significantly impaired.

Oestrogen receptors are found in liver tissue, and consequently the high levels of oestrogens contained in COCs that travel to the liver on first pass from the portal circulation may account for the number of hepatic complications associated with these preparations, e.g. cholestatic jaundice, hepatocellular carcinoma, Budd–Chiari syndrome [2].

The pharmacokinetics of hormonal contraceptives are likely to be affected by liver dysfunction, and this may have an impact on the efficacy of the drug or its side-effect profile.

Examples of factors which could reduce contraceptive levels:

- Enterohepatic circulation of EE may be affected by reduced biliary excretion in cholestasis, resulting in lower oestrogen levels.
- Cholestasis may decrease the absorption of fat-soluble drugs such as norgestimate and gestodene.
- Impaired metabolic capacity may reduce the conversion of drugs to active metabolites, e.g. desogestrel.
- The contraceptive efficacy of hormonal contraception (with the exception of the IMP or the LNG-IUD) is reduced by cytochrome P450 enzyme-inducing drugs.

Examples of factors which could increase contraceptive levels:

- Low albumin concentration could create higher levels of free contraceptive hormone in the blood. It is not know whether this higher free hormone has implications for liver patients.
- Cholestasis may reduce the elimination of gestodene through the biliary system.

There are a number of liver and non-liver medical contraindications to the use of contraceptives, and so each woman should have a full medical examination and medication history before a contraceptive method can be recommended. Patients should be assessed using the Faculty of Family Planning and Reproductive Health Care UK Medical Eligibility Criteria (FFPRHC UKMEC) [4].

The few trials of contraceptive methods in liver disease that have been performed are relatively old and do not necessarily correspond with the current guidance published by the World Health Organization (WHO) and FFPRHC in 2005/6.

Unless otherwise stated, all pharmacokinetic data originate from standard reference sources [5–10] and refer to adults.

Pharmacokinetics

See Table 13.1 for a summary of pharmacokinetic information relating to hormonal contraceptives.

Absorption

The oral bioavailability of many of these hormones is reduced because of first-pass metabolism; however, the parenteral routes, e.g. etonorgestrel (ENG) subdermal implant, provide almost 100% bioavailability. Gestodene and norgestimate are highly lipophilic and therefore absorption may be impaired in cholestasis. Medroxyprogesterone injection has a slow absorption from the injection site, which provides the product with its long duration of action [7, 11].

Distribution

Progestogens are all highly protein bound, primarily to sex hormone-binding globulin (SHBG), and to a lesser extent albumin. EE, on the other hand, is mainly bound to albumin, unlike naturally occurring oestrogens which are bound to SHBG. The proportion of levonorgestrel bound to SHBG increases when it is given with an oestrogen.

Hypoproteinaemia could increase the free fraction of these hormones [11].

Metabolism

EE and most progestogens undergo extensive first-pass metabolism in the liver and gut wall, reducing their oral bioavailability. To avoid first-pass metabolism progestogens and EE can be absorbed transdermally via the combined contraceptive patch. Some hormones are metabolised

Table 13.1 Pharmacokinetics of contraceptives

Drug	Oral bio-availability %	T_{max} (hrs)	Protein binding %	Half life (hrs)
Desogestrel	62–81	1.1–1.6	97.5	30
Ethinylestradiol	50 Although variable	1–2	>95	12
Gestodene	100	1.7	99.4	1.5
Levonorgestrel	90	1.6	93–95	16
Norethisterone	40	2	61	7.6
Norgestimate	Unknown	2	99	16.5
Medroxyprogesterone (Depo-Provera®)	–	3 weeks	94	6 weeks
Norethisterone (Noristerat®)	–	–	95	Biphasic release 4–5 days 15–20 days
Etonogestrel (Implanon®)	–	–	95.5–99	25
Levonorgestrel (Mirena®)	–	–	93–95	17
Ethinylestradiol and norelgestromin patch (Evra®)	–	Peak within 48		17 hours ethinyl estradiol and 28 hours norelgestromin

% excreted unchanged in urine	% Biliary excreted	Metabolism	Active metabolites
–	–	Hydroxylation followed by oxidation	Etonogestrel 3-hydroxydesogestrel
5–15	Approx 30	2-hydroxylation (CYP3A4) and sulphate and glucuronide conjugation and up to 30% is excreted unoxidized. Excretion is 60% renal and 40% in faeces. High first pass metabolism	Estrone (small amounts)
0	50	Reduction, oxidation and conjugation	
Very little	20–30	Reduction, hydroxylation and conjugation to form both sulfate and glucuronide conjugates	No
1	Partially via biliary route, % unknown	The major pathway is reduction then conjugation with sulfate or glucuronic acid and excretion in the urine High first-pass metabolism	
0	36.8 +/– 7.3	Hydrolysis	17-deacetyl norgestimate 3-ketonorgestimate levonorgestrel
5	–	Hyroxylation, de-esterification, transesterification Demethylation and reduction	
1	Partially via biliary route, % unknown	The major pathway is reduction then conjugation with sulfate or glucuronic acid and excretion in the urine	
–	–	Hydroxylation and reduction Metabolites are conjugated to sulfates and glucuronides	
Very little	20–30	Reduction, hydroxylation and conjugation to form both sulfate and glucuronide conjugates	No
	–		Norgestrel

to active metabolites, e.g. desogestrel is converted to the active metabolite ENG.

Elimination

Conjugates of EE, unaltered EE and progestogens are excreted into bile and released into the small intestine. Up to 30% of EE is excreted unoxidised in urine and bile. The sulphate and glucuronide conjugates of EE cannot be absorbed from the small intestine, but in the large intestine they are broken down by hydrolytic enzymes released from colonic bacteria (*Clostridia, Bacteroides* species, lactose-fermenting coliforms and some staphylococci) and reabsorbed. These active metabolites of EE are excreted in the urine [11]. The proportion of reabsorption of EE via the enterohepatic circulation can vary between patients. The relevance of this in relation to contraceptive efficacy is unclear, but it may be significant, especially if contraceptive pills are omitted. Women with a colectomy and ileostomy have no enterohepatic circulation of EE, but there is no reduction in COC efficacy in this situation. Progestogens do not undergo enterohepatic circulation [11].

Some relevant adverse effects

Hepatic effects

Adverse hepatic effects have been linked to the use of oral contraceptives, including hepatic dysfunction, cholestatic jaundice, benign hepatic tumours and peliosis hepatis. In addition, oral contraceptives have a number of less common but important effects on the liver. A correlation between the development of the Budd–Chiari syndrome and COCs has been described, and progestational derivatives have been linked to exacerbations of hepatic porphyria [12].

High-dose contraceptives were previously associated with jaundice and other hepatic complications, but with current lower-dose contraceptives this is no longer the case. Most women experience no adverse effects on liver function, but occasional hepatic changes can occur.

It has been debated whether women with a previous history of liver disease could take oral contraceptives when their LFTs have returned to normal with close monitoring. However, COCs should be avoided in women with a history of past or current benign or malignant hepatic tumours, active hepatitis, or familial defects of biliary excretion [13].

Cholestasis

Cholestatic jaundice is thought to occur in one out of every 10 000 oral contraceptive users. Jaundice generally appears within the first six cycles of use; however, one study of 38 patients suggested that symptoms appeared within the first three cycles, with the greatest number of reports being seen in the first cycle after the commencement of oral contraceptive agents. Non-specific symptoms such as anorexia, malaise and nausea often occurred for approximately two weeks prior to the identification of jaundice. The jaundice usually disappeared within a month after withdrawing the pill; however, if the patients were rechallenged jaundice and abnormal laboratory results reappeared. There were no long-term effects of note [14]. A number of familial liver disorders may be identified when a woman starts taking oral contraceptives; they include benign recurrent intrahepatic cholestasis, Dubin–Johnson syndrome and intrahepatic cholestasis of pregnancy [12].

Benign and malignant tumours

Hepatic adenomas, benign neoplasms consisting of hepatocytes, appear to be linked to the use of oral contraceptives, and before 1960 were rarely described. The incidence of hepatic adenomas has since increased, reflecting increased use of oral contraceptives, and in 1977 was estimated at five cases per million women aged 15–45 years. Hepatic adenomas have been detected in patients taking the pill continuously for a period of six months to four years [15]. To date, mestranol has been the constituent predominantly implicated [12].

The use of hormonal contraceptives for eight years or more has led to a 4.4-fold increased risk of hepatocellular carcinoma [24]. Such tumours develop in non-cirrhotic livers, and it has been found that they metastasise rarely and do not infiltrate [16]. There are limited data specifically on POCs. Results from a WHO study provided no evidence that use of DMPA altered the risk of developing liver cancer, but the power of the study to detect small alterations in risk was low [5].

Peliosis hepatis

Peliosis hepatis consists of a focal dilatation of the portal tract sinusoids. The condition is associated with contraceptive-induced hepatic tumours and can occasionally develop in isolation [13].

Hepatic venous outflow obstruction

The Budd–Chiari syndrome (BCS) is thought to be related to abnormal coagulation and is diagnosed by the identification of obstruction of large hepatic veins in the absence of tumour invasion or compression [15]. Oral contraceptives have been associated with an increased risk of BCS. It is thought that the oestrogen component of COCs is responsible [15]. Valla and colleagues [17], in a case–control study of 33 women with BCS, identified a relative risk of 2.37 for this complication in users of oral contraceptives, a figure very close to that for other vascular complications of the pill. Current evidence suggests that oral contraceptives lead to hepatic vein thrombosis by exacerbating an underlying thrombogenic condition [16].

Osteoporosis

DMPA has been found to reduce bone mineral density and increase the risk of osteoporosis or fractures in later life. Recent evidence states that DMPA causes a reduction in bone mineral density in adolescents [18]. As osteoporosis is a complication of some chronic liver diseases the potential reduction in bone mineral density should be considered before this method can be recommended.

Some relevant drug interactions

Drugs that induce cytochrome P450 (CYP3A4 is the major subtype) can reduce the efficacy of CHCs, POPs, and implants, but do not appear to reduce the efficacy of progestogen-only injectables or the LNG-IUD [11]. As the LNG-IUD has a local contraceptive action progestogenic interactions are less likely to occur. The efficacy of the contraceptive patch may be reduced by enzyme-inducing drugs [3, 11, 19].

Inhibition of cytochrome P450 enzymes is less relevant for women using hormonal contraceptives, as toxicity with EE or progestogens rarely occurs.

Some antibacterials that do not induce liver enzymes (e.g. ampicillin and doxycycline) have the potential to reduce the concentration of EE as a result of their effect on gut flora, which impairs enterohepatic circulation. Therefore, additional contraceptive methods should be advised for short courses (less than three weeks) as the efficacy of CHCs may be reduced [3, 11]. The efficacy of progestogen-only methods is not altered with non-liver-enzyme-inducing antibiotics, as progestogens are not dependent on enterohepatic circulation.

Clinical studies

Combined hormonal contraceptives

It is thought that oestrogens probably reduce bile-salt-independent bile flow through suppression of Na^+K^+-ATPase activity: consequently, liver plasma membranes become less fluid. Such changes in membrane fluidity are considered to be dose dependent [16]. It is therefore recommended that the combined oestrogen-formulated contraceptives should not be advocated for patients with CLD [1]. In particular, women with familial defects of biliary excretion, including Dubin–Johnson syndrome, Rotor's syndrome, and benign recurrent intrahepatic cholestasis, should avoid oestrogen-containing preparations. A reduction in hepatic excretory function induced by the oral contraceptive could convert mild hyperbilirubinaemia to jaundice [20].

The use of COCs in patients with Wilson's disease remains controversial. There are reports suggesting that COCs will increase plasma caeruloplasmin, leading to increased absorption of copper, and this could exacerbate the disease [21]. No data are available to evaluate this risk objectively. Patients should therefore use POCs [2].

In an open comparative trial of 156 women with compensated bilharzial liver disease (a condition consisting of hepatic features such as portal hypertension, ascites and haematemesis) with or without splenomegaly and with normal LFTs, Tagy [22] treated 38 women using a low-dose COC and 53 with depot medroxyprogesterone injections. There was no significant change in serum bilirubin, alkaline phosphatase or transaminases measured at either the first or the second follow-up visits in either arm compared to a control group of 65 women who used an intrauterine device (copper T380). The patients were followed for six months and all methods were found to be safe and effective.

Patients with acute hepatitis (hepatitis A, B, C or autoimmune hepatitis) are usually jaundiced with extremely elevated transaminases. COCs should not be used during the acute phase, as oestrogen derivatives could exacerbate hepatitis when combined with active inflammation of the liver [2]. One author stated that COCs should not be prescribed in a hepatitis A patient until three months after the LFTs have returned to normal [23].

Given that patients with chronic viral hepatitis are at risk for hepatocellular carcinoma (HCC), the use of COCs in these patients remains controversial. Some clinicians have suggested that COCs and chronic viral hepatitis may work synergistically to precipitate HCC. A specific link between HCC and combination oral contraceptives has not been established in this group of patients [2], but a study by Neuberger [24] highlighted an increased risk of HCC with COCs. He described a series of 26 women aged below 50 who developed HCC in a non-cirrhotic liver. These patients were studied for the possible role of COCs. Eighteen of them had used the pill for a median of eight years. Patients and controls were divided into five age and four calendar groups and the relative risks associated with oral contraceptives were calculated by multivariate analysis. Neuberger suggested that short-term use of the pill was not associated with an increased risk of tumour development; however, use for eight years or more was associated with a 4.4-fold increased risk (p < 0.01) [24].

Cholestasis of pregnancy appears to be stimulated by the high oestrogen concentrations present at the time [25]. Kreek [26] identified cholestatic jaundice in a patient that recurred during each subsequent pregnancy, with liver biopsies showing intrahepatic cholestasis. When the patient was challenged with oral EE the clinical symptoms of jaundice and abnormal LFTs returned, suggesting that cholestasis of pregnancy may have a hormonal basis [26]. Historically, it was considered that women with cholestasis of pregnancy have a 50% chance of acquiring cholestasis while on COCs [26], and therefore they should consider POCs or barrier methods as their first choice of contraception. If the CHC method is to be proposed in a patient with a previous history of pregnancy-related cholestasis it is advisable to consider the patient's current hepatic function, as the method should be deferred until the LFTs have returned to normal. After initiation of the CHC the patient should be monitored for any symptoms of jaundice or changes in LFTs for the first six contraceptive cycles.

Orellana-Alcalde et al. [14] postulated a link between the use of progestogen- and oestrogen-containing contraceptives and cholestatic jaundice with severe pruritus. Fifty patients who had developed jaundice and pruritus while taking oral contraceptives were investigated. All other possible types of jaundice had been excluded. The contraceptive agents that had been taken were norethynodrel or lynoestrenol as the progestogen, and ethinylestradiol or mestranol as the oestrogen. Seventeen patients had experienced pruritus and jaundice during previous pregnancies. Ten patients had experienced late pruritus of a previous pregnancy. In 26 patients the symptoms appeared within the first contraceptive cycle. The clinical and biochemical findings in the study patients bore a strong resemblance to those of intrahepatic cholestasis of pregnancy. When the contraceptive method was withdrawn, the pruritus and jaundice disappeared within seven to 60 days. The authors suggested that jaundice due to such oral contraceptives could have a similar aetiological basis to cholestatic jaundice of pregnancy, because a number of the subjects previously had jaundice and pruritus during pregnancy [14]. This study did not specify which agent, oestrogen or progestogen, caused the pruritus and jaundice, therefore we have to assume that both agents could precipitate this condition.

Weden [27] described a protracted cholestasis which was thought to be induced by the use of a COC. The patient's liver biopsy revealed changes including eosinophilia and sinusoidal dilatation, which could be linked to a drug-induced liver injury. The cholestasis gradually disappeared, but an elevated serum alkaline phosphatase level continued for up to ten years after discontinuation of the COC [27]. Another paper has discussed oestrogen-induced cholestasis and highlights the link between the use of COCs and intrahepatic cholestasis [28].

A review of 253 cases of Budd–Chiari syndrome found COC use to be the presumed cause in 9% of patients [29]. There appears to be a correlation between the development of BCS and the oestrogenic component of COCs [12]. Obstruction of the hepatic and portal veins has been documented and has been attributed to the thrombotic effects of the COCs; however, the affected women may have had an underlying coagulation defect [16]. Budd–Chiari patients should be advised not to use COCs, as such patients have a demonstrated haematological tendency to form thrombi, and oestrogen-containing contraceptives may increase the risk of recurrent thrombosis [2].

It is important to highlight the current FFPRHC UK Medical Eligibility Criteria (UKMEC) guidance (adapted from WHO) relating to the use of CHCs in patients with liver disease, as this information may differ from the clinical studies outlined above:

- Pregnancy-related cholestasis – category 2 advantages outweigh the risks.
- Past COC-related cholestasis – category 3 risks outweigh the advantages.
- Active viral hepatitis – category 4 unacceptable health risk if method is used.
- Carrier hepatitis – category 1 no restriction for use of the method.
- Compensated cirrhosis – category 3 risks outweigh the advantages.

- Decompensated cirrhosis – category 4 unacceptable health risk if method is used.
- Adenoma – category 4 unacceptable health risk if method is used.
- Hepatoma – category 4 unacceptable health risk if method is used.

Progestogen-only contraceptives (POCs)

It is thought that progesterone derivatives have the least effect on liver metabolism and provide a reliable assurance against pregnancy. Hepatic disturbance is not considered a contraindication to progesterone therapy [2], but in practice the method cannot be recommended in active viral hepatitis or severe decompensated cirrhosis [4]. Viral hepatitis carriers can use the POC methods in any circumstance [30]. When patients with acute hepatitis recover fully and LFTs have returned to normal, the full spectrum of contraceptive choices can be considered; however, such patients should be monitored carefully during the initiation period [2].

A small historical study evaluated the effect of DMPA on six patients with either chronic active viral hepatitis or primary biliary cirrhosis. The study showed that DMPA actually improved transaminase levels and the metabolic ability of the liver. The investigators suggested that the immune-modifying properties of medroxyprogesterone may make the hormone a therapeutic alternative [2]. There were limitations in that this was a very small, non-randomised study, and therefore it is difficult to make specific recommendations based on the outcome. Another study of the metabolic effects of DMPA in women who had used the method for five years or more suggested that there was a significant rise in plasma insulin, alkaline phosphatase and morning cortisol levels in the DMPA users [31].

The Tagy study discussed earlier [22] showed DMPA to be safe in compensated bilharzial liver fibrosis, although this could be difficult to extrapolate to other liver diseases.

Again, the current FFPRHC UKMEC guidance relating to the use of POCs in patients with liver disease differs in places from the clinical studies outlined above:

- Pregnancy-related cholestasis – category 1 no restriction for the use of the method.
- Past COC-related cholestasis – category 2 advantages outweigh the risks.
- Active viral hepatitis – category 3 risks outweigh the advantages.
- Carrier hepatitis – category 1 no restriction for the use of the method.
- Compensated cirrhosis – category 2 advantages outweigh the risks.

- Decompensated cirrhosis – category 3 risks outweigh the advantages.
- Adenoma – category 3 risks outweigh the advantages.
- Hepatoma – category 3 risks outweigh the advantages.

Intrauterine devices (IUDs)

The use of IUDs in patients with CLD has complicating factors. Owing to reduced hepatic complement synthesis and reticuloendothelial system dysfunction, patients with cirrhosis and ascites are prone to develop repeated episodes of spontaneous bacterial peritonitis (SBP). Historically, the risk of pelvic inflammatory disease (PID) was considered to be increased in IUD users during the first year after insertion, therefore it was thought that the presence of an IUD in approximation with the peritoneal surface in a patient with cirrhotic ascites might lead to SBP [1]. Farley et al. [32] recognised that earlier studies suggested that infection rates from IUD insertion were found to be initially high, then fell away and remained constant in later months, hence some guidance still states that infection can occur up to one year after insertion. The Farley study found that the highest infection risk was noted to be in the first 20 days after insertion. They also found that IUDs did not increase infection risk with long-term use. The group identified a higher risk of infection immediately after insertion, but that the risk could possibly be minimised by prophylactic antibiotics given at the time of insertion [32]. The current FFPRHC advice suggests that LNG-IUDs and Cu-IUD can be considered in patients with compensated cirrhosis [4]. When considering either the LNG-IUD or the Cu- IUD methods the patient should be assessed to identify whether their liver disease could make them prone to infection [7]. If the patient selects the IUD method, the need for prophylactic antibiotics at the time of insertion should be considered.

IUD use can cause excessive uterine bleeding owing to its local effect on the endometrium [7]. Excessive uterine bleeding can endanger cirrhotic patients with a pre-existing bleeding tendency [1]. This risk is not addressed in the FFPRHC guidance, and therefore caution is advised when recommending IUDs in cirrhotic patients as they invariably have coagulopathy. The LNG-IUD is not recommended in decompensated cirrhosis; however, the Cu-IUD could be considered [4]. Coagulation disturbances are deemed a contraindication to insertion of an IUD, and so a coagulation screen is advisable before recommending the method [7].

Wilson's disease is characterised by a malfunction in the ability of the liver to excrete copper. Speroff et al. [33] stated that the additional copper load of copper-based IUDs could theoretically exacerbate

Wilson's disease, and therefore they suggested that it be contraindicated in such patients. The Nova T 380 device, which is a copper-based IUD licensed in the UK, is now contraindicated in Wilson's disease [7].

It is thought that the contraceptive needs of hepatitis patients and patients with active liver disease are better met with an IUD, as all oral hormonal methods should be avoided [2, 34]. The Cu-IUD is a good choice for women with active viral hepatitis [35]. The FFPRHC believe that in active viral hepatitis the theoretical or proven risks usually outweigh the advantages of using the LNG-IUD [4], therefore the copper-containing IUD would be the IUD of choice in this situation. Viral hepatitis carriers can use both IUD methods (Cu and LNG) [30].

The FFPRHC have advised that the IUD method can be advocated in pregnancy-related cholestasis. Both Cu and LNG IUDs can be used [4, 30]. There is concern that a history of COC-related cholestasis may predict subsequent cholestasis with the LNG-IUD; however, as the device has a local effect the risk of side-effects is thought to be minimal, and there are no trial data to support or contradict this concern [30]. However, because of the theoretical risk it would be advisable to monitor LFTs after the insertion of a LNG-IUD.

IUDs appear to be safe in patients with Budd–Chiari syndrome [2] unless there is significant ascites, a substantial infection risk, or coagulation abnormalities that could precipitate haemorrhage after insertion.

Barrier methods

Condoms should be recommended to infectious patients to prevent the spread of viral hepatitis [31]. In all other liver diseases the barrier method provides an ideal non-hormonal option for contraception.

CASE STUDIES

See Appendix 1 for full details of the following patient cases.

Patient 1 – Mild hepatitis without cirrhosis

The synthetic and metabolic capacity of this patient's liver is unlikely to be affected by the isolated rise in ALT, and drug handling is unlikely to be altered. It is important to ensure that the patient has no signs of cirrhosis, as many diseases that present with this clinical picture can be cirrhotic despite near-normal laboratory tests.

- CHCs should be avoided as they may exacerbate the hepatitis.

- This patient's obesity would also contraindicate CHCs, which should generally be avoided in women with a body mass index >35 kg/m².
- POCs could be used in this patient as the liver disease is mild, with normal hepatocyte function. LFTs should be monitored to ensure the hepatitis is not aggravated.
- Both autoimmune and viral hepatitis, which could present with a similar clinical picture to patient 1, are contraindications to the use of POCs as they could worsen the clinical course.
- IUDs would be appropriate, although if the LNG-IUD was chosen then LFTs should be monitored after insertion to ensure that no deterioration in liver function occurred.
- Barrier methods would be a suitable option, with no side effects. However, the lower efficacy rate would need to be considered, as fertility in this patient is likely to be normal.

Patient 2 – Cholestasis

The synthetic and metabolic capacity of this patient's liver is unlikely to be affected by cholestasis. However, consideration needs to be given to protein binding (patient has hyperbilirubinaemia); excretion of the drug or metabolites in bile (patient has cholestasis); and the lipophilicity of the drug (some lipophilic drugs require bile salts for absorption and these would be reduced in cholestasis).

- There is evidence that pre-existing cholestasis increases the risk of jaundice and pruritus with hormonal contraceptives; consequently, CHCs and probably POCs would be contraindicated in this patient.
- The pharmacokinetics of hormonal contraception would also be affected by cholestasis:
    - Reduced enterohepatic circulation of EE, potentially reducing contraceptive efficacy
    - Reduced absorption of the lipophilic drugs (gestodene and norgestimate)
    - Reduced biliary excretion of EE, gestogen and norgestimate.
- The drug interactions with rifampicin and ciprofloxacin would also need to be taken into account if hormonal methods were used [19, 36].
- IUDs could be used in cholestatic patients, with the Cu-IUD as first choice to minimise any potential progestogen challenge. However, in this patient there is a history of recurrent cholangitis infections, and this may increase the risk of insertion-related infection. It should only be contemplated if she has been infection free for some time, and prophylactic antibiotics should be considered at insertion. The clotting should be checked before insertion as it could be reduced secondary to vitamin K malabsorption.
- Barrier methods would be safe in this patient.

Patient 3 – Compensated cirrhosis

Despite cirrhosis, this patient is maintaining good hepatocyte function (normal albumin and bilirubin, mildly raised INR) and the metabolic and excretory capacity of the liver should not be significantly reduced. The patient has portal hypertension, so blood flow to the liver will be impaired, which will reduce first-pass metabolism of highly extracted drugs (extraction ratio >0.7). This will result in greater bioavailability of oral doses of these drugs. It is important to note that the patient could rapidly deteriorate into a state of decompensation where liver function would be markedly affected.

Other things to consider are the raised INR and low platelet count (avoid drugs that affect coagulation or cause bleeding), the risk of encephalopathy if the liver function decompensates, and the risk of hepatorenal syndrome.

- As hepatic disturbance is not considered a contraindication to POCs this method could be used with caution in mildly cirrhotic patients. Routine LFTs should be performed to monitor for decompensation after initiation. Barrier methods such as condoms could also be considered.
- This patient has a low platelet count and a raised INR, therefore the insertion of an IUD could put her at risk of excessive intrauterine bleeding and cannot be recommended.
- The use of CHCs could accelerate decompensation owing to the hormone burden on the liver, and therefore they cannot be recommended.

Patient 4 – Decompensated cirrhosis

This patient has decompensated liver disease with significantly impaired synthetic, metabolic and excretory function (low albumin, raised INR, hyperbilirubinaemia, encephalopathy). The reduction in hepatocyte mass and function will significantly reduce the metabolism of low extraction ratio drugs (hepatocyte dependent). The patient also has severe portal hypertension, which will reduce first-pass metabolism, increasing the bioavailability of high extraction ratio drugs. The ascites may affect the absorption of some drugs and may alter the distribution of hydrophilic drugs. Highly protein-bound drugs may be affected by hypoalbuminaemia and hyperbilirubinaemia, resulting in increased levels of free drug. The cholestasis may impair oral absorption of lipid-soluble drugs and may also reduce biliary excretion.

Conception and pregnancy would be unlikely in CLD. When considering contraceptive methods for this patient it is important to address her current medical conditions, including episodes of SBP requiring non-enzyme inducing antibiotics that could affect the gut flora, ascites, and pre-existing bleeding tendencies.

- Barrier methods such as condoms would be the most appropriate choice in this situation.
- As this patient has decompensated cirrhosis with ascites and a documented history of repeated episodes of SBP, an IUD cannot be considered as this method is contraindicated in patients prone to infection and experiencing disorders of coagulation.
- As CHCs and POCs are metabolised by the liver their use may adversely affect this patient, who has severely compromised liver function. CHC or POC methods should not be advocated in this case. This patient's synthetic and metabolic function is significantly impaired and therefore the metabolism of CHCs could be affected, precipitating adverse drug reactions such as jaundice, hepatitis and cholestasis.

Patient 5 – Acute liver failure

As this patient is acutely unwell contraception would not be an immediate issue. It may be important to consider in the future, depending on the clinical course.

If this patient is using an IUD at the time of the acute episode, its removal should be considered to reduce the risk of intrauterine bleeding. Prophylactic antibiotics should be recommended before the removal procedure [7].

Acknowledgements

I would like to thank Dr Astrid Scalori, Specialist Hepatology Registrar, and Dr Usha Kumar, Family Planning Consultant, King's College Hospital, London, for their comments during the preparation of this chapter.

References

1. Haimov-Kochman R, Ackerman Z, Anteby EY (1997) The contraceptive choice for a Wilson's disease patient with chronic liver disease. *Contraception* 56: 241–244.
2. Connolly TJ, Zuckerman AL (1998) Contraception in the patient with liver disease. *Semin Perinatol* 22: 178–182.
3. British Medical Association and Royal Pharmaceutical Society of Great Britain (2006) *British National Formulary* No 52. London: BMJ Publishing Group Ltd and Pharmaceutical Press.

4. Faculty of Family Planning and Reproductive Health Care (2006) UK Medical Eligibility Criteria for Contraceptive Use (UKMEC 2005/2006). London: Faculty of Family Planning and Reproductive Health Care.

5. Sweetman SC (ed) (2002) *Martindale. The Complete Drug Reference,* 33rd edn. London: Pharmaceutical Press, 1527–1536.

6. McEvoy GK (ed) (1995) *American Hospital Formulary Service Drug Information.* Bethesda, MD: American Society of Health-System Pharmacists.

7. Electronic Medicines Compendium. Datapharm Communications Ltd. http://emc.medicines.org.uk/ (last accessed 9 March 2007).

8. Trissel LA (2003) *Handbook on Injectable Drugs,* 12th edn. Bethesda, MD: American Society of Health-System Pharmacists.

9. Thomson Healthcare Products. Micromedex Healthcare Series. http://www.thomsonhc.com (last accessed 9 March 2007).

10. Dollery C (ed) (1999) *Therapeutic Drugs,* 2nd edn. Edinburgh: Churchill Livingstone.

11. Faculty of Family Planning and Reproductive Health Care Clinical Effectiveness Unit (2005) FFPRHC Guidance: Drug Interactions with Hormonal Contraception. *J Fam Plan Health Care* 31: 139–150.

12. Lockhat D, Katz SS, Lisbona R, Mishkin S (1981) Oral contraceptives and liver disease. *CMAJ* 124: 993–999.

13. Aronson JK (ed) (2006) *Meyler's Side Effects of Drugs,* 15th edn. Amsterdam: Elsevier.

14. Orellana-Alcalde JM, Dominguez JP (1966) Jaundice and oral contraceptive drugs. *Lancet* 2: 1278–1280.

15. Farrell GC (1994) *Drug-Induced Liver Disease.* Melbourne: Churchill Livingstone.

16. Sherlock S (1986) The spectrum of hepatotoxicity due to drugs. *Lancet* 2: 440–444.

17. Valla D, Le MG, Paynard T, Rueff B, Benhamou JP (1986) Risk of hepatic vein thrombosis in relation to the recent use of oral contraceptives: a case control study. *Gastroenterology* 90: 967–972.

18. National Prescribing Centre (2006) Contraception – current issues. *MeReC Bull* 17: 2.

19. Gupta KC, Ali MY (1980) Failure of oral contraceptive with rifampicin. *Med J Zambia* 15: 23.

20. Lindberg MC (1992) Hepatobiliary complications of oral contraceptives. *J Gen Intern Med* 7: 199–209.

21. Decherney AH (1981) The use of birth control pills in women with medical disorders. *Clin Obstet Gynecol* 24: 965–975.

22. Tagy A, Saker M, Moussa A, Kolgah A (2001) The effect of low dose combined oral contraceptive pills versus injectable contraceptive (Depot Provera) on liver function tests of women with compensated bilharzial liver fibrosis. *Contraception* 64: 173–176.

23. Rowlands S (1991) Contrasting contraceptive needs. *Practitioner* 235: 868–873.

24. Neuberger J, Forman D, Doll R, Williams R (1986) Oral contraceptives and hepatocellular carcinoma. *Br Med J* 292: 1355–1357.

25. Cunningham FG, Leveno KJ (1993) *Williams Obstetrics*, 19th edn. Norwalk, CT: Appleton & Lange.

26. Kreek MJ, Sleisenger MH, Jeffries GH (1967) Recurrent cholestatic jaundice of pregnancy with demonstrated oestrogen sensitivity. *Am J Med* 43: 79–203.

27. Weden M, Glaumann H, Einarsson K (1992) Protracted cholestasis probably induced by oral contraceptive. J Intern Med 231: 561–565.

28. Schreiber AJ, Simon FR (1983) Estrogen-induced cholestasis: clues to pathogenesis and treatment. *Hepatology* 3: 607–613.

29. Mitchell MC, Boitnott JK, Kaufman S (1982) Budd–Chiari syndrome: Etiology, diagnosis and management. *Medicine* 61: 199–218.

30. World Health Organization (2004) *Improving Access to Quality Care in Family Planning. Medical Eligibility Criteria for Contraceptive Use*, 3rd edn. Geneva: Reproductive Health and Research World Health Organization.

31. Virutamasen P, Wongsrichanalai C, Tangkeo P, Nitchai Y, Rienprayonn D (1986) Metabolic effects of depot-medroxyprogesterone acetate in long-term users: a cross-sectional study. *Int J Gynaecol Obstet* 24: 291–296.

32. Farley TMM, Rosenberg MJ, Rowe PJ, Chien JH, Meirik O (1992) Intrauterine devices and pelvic inflammatory disease: an international perspective. *Lancet* 339: 785–788.

33. Speroff L, Darney PD (1992) *A Clinical Guide for Contraception*. Baltimore, MD: Williams & Wilkins.

34. Nelson AL (1998) Intrauterine device practice guidelines: medical conditions. *Contraception* 58: 59S–63S.

35. Chronic Diseases and Contraceptive Use (1999) Network 19(2): 14–15.

36. Scholten PC, Droppert RM, Zwinkels MGL, Moesker HL, Nauta JJP, Hoepelman IM (1998) No interaction between ciprofloxacin and an oral contraceptive. *Antimicrob Agents Chemother* 42: 3266–3268.

Appendix 1

Detailed description of the five patient cases

Patient 1 – Mild hepatitis without cirrhosis

Patient details

Patient 1 is an obese 45-year-old with raised transaminases which were discovered on admission to hospital with a chest infection. There is no past medical history or drug history of note. Investigations were undertaken for hepatitis.

Diagnosis

Non-alcoholic steatohepatitis

Medication history

None at time of presentation

Signs and symptoms

Occasional abdominal pain
No stigmata of chronic liver disease

Blood results

Test	(normal range)	Result – trend: ↑ ↓ ↔
ALT	(<40 IU/L)	146 ↑
Bilirubin	(5–21 µmol/L)	7 ↔
Alk phos	(70–300 IU/L)	256 ↔
GGT	(<40 IU/L)	43 ↔
Albumin	(34–48 g/L)	45 ↔
INR	(0.9–1.2)	1.2 ↔
Creatinine	(70–100 µmol/L)	79 ↔

Other tests

Ultrasound – large liver with fatty infiltration
Liver biopsy – steatosis, mild steatohepatitis and fibrosis. Normal liver architecture, no cholestasis, severely fatty liver

Possible alternative diagnoses

Drug side effect (i.e. transient raised transaminases)/toxicity
Viral hepatitis (usually much higher transaminases) – acute or chronic
Autoimmune hepatitis
α_1-antitrypsin deficiency
Coeliac disease
Muscle disease
Alcoholic liver disease
Sepsis

Summary of liver function and drug handling

The raised ALT suggests there is some ongoing hepatocyte damage; however, there are no other biochemical markers of liver disease. This probably reflects mild disease, confirmed by a lack of signs or symptoms of chronic liver disease, with no cirrhosis on biopsy. The liver has normal synthetic function (normal INR and albumin), no evidence of cholestasis and only mildly raised transaminases. It is to be expected that the hepatocytes would be able to maintain their normal metabolic function and that drug handling would be unaffected in this patient. It is important to confirm that a patient with a similar picture of LFTs is not cirrhotic, as this would affect metabolism and drug handling.

Patient 2 – Cholestasis

Patient details

Patient 2, a 65-year-old, presented two years ago with a flu-like illness associated with fever and rigors. Jaundice and abnormal liver enzymes subsequently developed, and further investigations strongly suggested a diagnosis of primary sclerosing cholangitis (PSC). Patient 2 had significant problems with itching and recurrent cholangitis.

Diagnosis

Primary sclerosing cholangitis.

Medication history

Rifampicin – for pruritus
Ursodeoxycholic acid – to improve bile flow
Ciprofloxacin – for recurrent cholangitis
Vitamins A and D – fat-soluble vitamin supplements

Signs and symptoms

Jaundice
Pruritus
No obvious signs of chronic liver disease, e.g. portal hypertension, varices, ascites

Blood results

Test	(normal range)	Result – trend: ↑ ↓ ↔
ALT	(<40 IU/L)	60 ↔
Bilirubin	(5–21 µmol/L)	55 ↔
Alk phos	(70–300 IU/L)	1646 ↑
Albumin	(34–48 g/L)	40 ↔
INR/	(0.9–1.2)	1.0 ↔
PT	(9–15 seconds)	12 ↔
Creatinine/	(80–115 µmol/L)	100 ↔
creatinine clearance	(mL/min)	65 ↔

Other tests

ERCP – intra- and extrahepatic PSC
ANCA positive, other autoantibodies negative
Liver biopsy consistent with PSC
MRI scan – no evidence of tumour

Possible alternative diagnoses

Obstructive jaundice, e.g. gallstones/cholangiocarcinoma/other infiltration
Primary biliary cirrhosis
Drugs/toxins
Cholangitis
Autoimmune hepatitis

Summary of liver function and drug handling

This patient shows a cholestatic picture with a raised bilirubin and alkaline phosphatase. In terms of drug handling this may cause reduced absorption of some lipid-soluble drugs and impaired elimination of biliary excreted drugs. The ALT is raised but synthetic function is maintained, as indicated by a normal INR and albumin. This suggests that the hepatocytes are working effectively and therefore the metabolic function of the liver is unlikely to be altered in this patient.

Patient 3 – Compensated cirrhosis

Patient details

Patient 3, a 14-year-old, has a two-and-a-half-year history of chronic liver disease, which initially presented with severe abdominal pain. There have been no further problems, and apart from hospital admissions for investigations, patient 3 has been fit and well.

Diagnosis

Cryptogenic cirrhosis
MELD score 10 (NB: PELD <12 years)

Medication history

None

Signs and symptoms

Portal hypertension with a single oesophageal varix – grade 1, no history of bleeding
Spider naevi
Occasional tiredness
Occasional abdominal pain
Splenomegaly

Blood results

Test	(normal range)	Result – trend: ↑ ↓ ↔
ALT	(<40 IU/L)	60 ↔
Bilirubin	(5–21 µmol/L)	15 ↔
Alk phos	(70–600 IU/L – adolescent range)	547 ↔
GGT	(<40 IU/L)	23 ↔
Albumin	(34–48 g/L)	36 ↔
INR	(0.8–1.2)	1.4 ↔
Creatinine	(60–100 µmol /L – adolescent range)	51 ↔
Platelets	(150–400 × 10⁹/L)	75 ↔

Other tests

Ultrasound – abnormal heterogeneous texture to the liver; enlarged spleen (19 cm)
Endoscopy – single grade 1 varix and single fundal varix
Liver biopsy – established cryptogenic cirrhosis (inactive). No cholestasis or interface hepatitis

Possible alternative diagnoses

Autoimmune hepatitis
Chronic viral hepatitis
Non-alcoholic steatohepatitis (NASH)
Wilson's disease
α_1-antitrypsin disease
Metabolic/inherited diseases
Drugs/toxins
Alcoholic cirrhosis
ANY FORM OF LIVER DISEASE CAUSING CIRRHOSIS

Summary of liver function and drug handling

This patient has only a mildly raised ALT; however, the biopsy shows cirrhosis, and with the signs and symptoms of chronic liver disease (portal hypertension, splenomegaly, varices, spider naevi) this suggests there will be marked hepatocyte damage. Despite this, the liver is still managing to maintain its synthetic function (normal albumin, slightly raised INR) and excretory function (normal bilirubin). As the patient is well compensated the metabolic capacity of the liver should not be significantly impaired. However, it is important to note that a compensated cirrhotic patient can rapidly deteriorate to a decompensated state. As this patient has portal hypertension the metabolism of high extraction drugs is likely to be affected due to reduced blood flow through the liver, leading to higher oral bioavailability of the drug. Other drug handling parameters, e.g. protein binding and biliary excretion, should remain unaffected in this patient.

Patient 4 – Decompensated cirrhosis

Patient details

Patient 4 is a 58-year-old with a history of excess alcohol intake: approximately 60 units per week for the past four years. Recent admissions have been for ascites requiring paracentesis, spontaneous bacterial peritonitis, and large variceal bleeds. Over the last six months the patient has had a reduced appetite, poor nutrition and a significant loss of muscle mass.

Diagnosis

Alcoholic liver disease
Child–Pugh score C/MELD score 25

Medication history

Spironolactone – for ascites
Menadiol (vitamin K) – for coagulopathy
Propranolol – to reduce portal pressure
Vitamin B Co strong/thiamine – supplements
Ciprofloxacin – spontaneous bacterial peritonitis prophylaxis

Signs and symptoms

Ascites
Portal hypertension with varices, two previous bleeds
Encephalopathy grade II
Spider naevi
Weight loss over past six months
Jaundice

Blood results

Test	(normal range)	Result – trend: ↑ ↓ ↔
ALT	(<40 IU/L)	49 ↔
Bilirubin	(5–21 µmol/L)	180 ↑
Alk phos	(70–300 IU/L)	328 ↔
Albumin	(34–48 g/L)	28 ↓
INR/	(0.9–1.2)	1.6 ↑
PT	(9–15 seconds)	20 ↑
Creatinine/	(80–115 µmol/L)	138 ↔
creatinine clearance	(mL/min)	54 ↔

Other tests

Ultrasound – normal spleen, small nodular liver, ascites
Doppler – patent portal vein
Biopsy – cirrhosis

Possible alternative diagnoses

Cryptogenic cirrhosis
Chronic viral hepatitis
Non-alcoholic steatohepatitis (NASH)
Autoimmune hepatitis
Wilson's disease
α_1-antitrypsin disease
Metabolic/inherited diseases
Drugs/toxins
ANY FORM OF LIVER DISEASE CAUSING CIRRHOSIS

Summary of liver function and drug handling

The ALT is only slightly raised in this patient, but the other LFTs indicate that the liver's synthetic, metabolic and excretory function is significantly impaired (raised INR despite vitamin K, low albumin, raised bilirubin and encephalopathy) and that he has decompensated cirrhosis. This will affect the metabolism of low extraction ratio drugs. Patient 4 also has portal hypertension, and this will impair drug handling of high extraction ratio drugs, increasing their oral bioavailability. The changes will result in a greater area under the curve for most hepatically metabolised drugs and accumulation. The cholestasis and ascites may impair oral absorption of some drugs; ascites and low albumin may affect the distribution of hydrophilic and highly protein-bound drugs, respectively; and cholestasis may impair biliary excretion. This patient also appears to be developing some renal impairment, possibly hepatorenal syndrome, which will affect the excretion of renally excreted drugs. The calculated creatinine clearance is probably an overestimate of actual renal function.

Patient 5 – Acute liver failure

Patient details

Patient 5 is a 16-year-old who took a paracetamol overdose, consisting of 30 × 500 mg tablets, after an argument with parents. The patient presented to Accident and Emergency two days later with severe abdominal pain and vomiting.

Diagnosis

Paracetamol overdose

Medication history

Nil

Signs and symptoms

Encephalopathy grade III
Nausea
Vomiting
Abdominal pain
Jaundice
No evidence of chronic liver disease

Blood results

Test	(normal range)	Result – trend: ↑ ↑ ↔
ALT	(<40 IU/L)	13 078 ↑↑
Bilirubin	(5–21 µmol/L)	66 ↑
Alk phos	(70–300 IU/L)	245 ↑
Albumin	(34–48 g/L)	38 ↔
INR	(0.9–1.2)	5.3 ↑
Creatinine	(60–100 µmol/L – adolescent range)	190 ↑
creatinine clearance	(mL/min)	41 ↓

Other tests

Hepatitis screen – negative
Autoantibody screen – negative

Possible alternative diagnoses

Acute viral hepatitis
Other drugs/toxins
Metabolic disorders
Hypoxia/ischaemia

Summary of liver function and drug handling

This patient has a massively raised ALT, indicating considerable hepatocyte damage. All functions of the liver are likely to be affected, including reduced secretory and excretory function, demonstrated in this case by a raised bilirubin; reduced synthetic function, shown by the raised INR (albumin is unaffected at this time due to its long half life); reduced metabolic function, indicated by accumulation of ammonia and other toxins leading to encephalopathy. Blood flow through the liver is likely to be unaffected, as there is no cirrhosis/portal hypertension. As with all other functions of the liver, this patient's ability to metabolise drugs is likely to be severely affected. Renal function is also impaired secondary to paracetamol toxicity.

Appendix 2

Drugs in liver dysfunction –
blank *aide mémoire* form

Patient information

Name/DoB/unit number: _____

Diagnosis (type/cause)(if known): _____

Relevant biochemical tests: _____

Test	Result – recent changes $\uparrow \downarrow \leftrightarrow$	Normal range
ALT/AST		
Bilirubin		
Split bilirubin*		
Alk phos		
GGT		
Albumin		
INR/PT		
Creatinine/creatinine clearance/GFR**		

Caution: Check for non-liver causes of abnormal results e.g. warfarin, bone disease.
* May be useful in determining reason for hyperbilirubinaemia – not a routine test.
** Caution with interpreting in cirrhotic patients.

Signs of liver disease and useful test results likely to have an impact on drug handling

Sign	Present?	Tests	Result
Gynaecomastia		Biopsy	
Ascites		ERCP/HIDA	
Varices		Ultrasound scan – Doppler	
Failure to thrive weight loss		Endoscopy	
Pale stools		MELD/PELD/ Childs Pugh	
Encephalopathy		Encephalopathy score/grade	

Using all the information available, including the signs and test results, tick which apply with severity or grade if known.

Effect on kinetics/dynamics		Risk factors for side effects	
Ascites (A/D)		Varices	
Cholestasis (A/E)		Coagulopathy or low platelets	
Low albumin (D)		Encephalopathy	
Portal hypertension (M)		Pruritus	
Acute liver failure (M)		Alcoholism	
Cirrhosis – compensated (M)		Ascites	
Cirrhosis – decompensated (M)		Renal impairment/hepatorenal	
Encephalopathy (P)		Cirrhosis	

A: Absorption;   D: Distribution;   M: Metabolism;   E: Elimination;   P: Pharmacodynamics

Drug considerations

Drug . . . .

Pharmacokinetics

		Considerations
Absorption		Lipid solubility (absorption affected by ascites)
Distribution		Water/fat Protein binding % Displaced by bilirubin or displaces bilirubin
Metabolism		First-pass effect Hepatocyte dependent Prodrug CYPs Active metabolites Genetics
Elimination		Biliary excretion Alternative mechanisms Enterohepatic recirculation (renal impairment)

Side effects
Consider: GI ulceration, sedation, coagulopathy, platelet effects, effects on fluid balance, effect on electrolytes, biliary sludging, renal impairment, constipation

Hepatotoxicity – known hepatotoxin/type

Published information in specific liver diseases/clinical studies
BNF/SPC

Concomitant drug interactions and other patient considerations, e.g. age, renal function, contraindications

Summary/answer

Index

Note: page numbers in *italics* refer to figures and tables